A HANDBOOK OF HY

A PRACTITIONERS' GUIDE

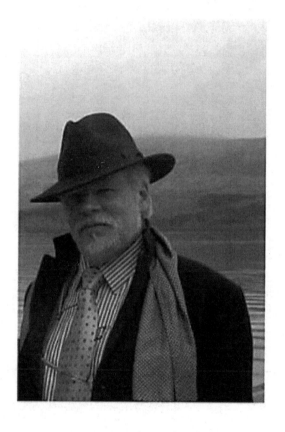

Peter Marshall

Key To Books

PROFESSIONAL-DEVELOPMENT

A HANDBOOK OF HYPNOTHERAPY

A practitioner's guide

Dr Peter Marshall

Key To Books

British Library Cataloguing in Publication Data
A catalogue record of this book is available from the British Library.

© Copyright 2012 by Peter Marshall.

Published by Key To Books 2012.

Reprinted 2017.

Key To Books is an imprint of Oakley Books Ltd., 10 Buckhurst Road, Bexhill on Sea, East Sussex, TN40 1QF.

Note: the material contained in this book is set out in good faith for general guidance and no liability can be accepted for loss or expense incurred as a result of relying in particular circumstances on statements made in the book. The laws and regulations are complex and liable to change and readers should check the current position with the relevant authorities before making personal arrangements.

Cover design by Pentacor Design.
Printed and bound in Exeter by Imprint Digital.

Contents

Preface

PREFACE

Hypnotism is a fascinating subject. Although it is, perhaps, most readily associated in the layperson's eyes with stage acts, its most important use is in therapy, where it is a powerful tool for bringing about rapid correction of disorders due to maladaptation. It is, for example, powerful in curing addictions, such as the smoking habit, phobias, lack of confidence, low self-esteem, performance anxiety and many more conditions.

There are many books on the subject, but most are general theoretical works. Others deal with specific therapies, such as phobias or smoking addiction. There are hardly any handbooks for practitioners. What there are mainly tend to represent the American approach and are not readily available in the UK bookshops. Consequently, hypnotism schools in the UK are unable to prescribe a set textbook. This book is intended to fill that gap in the market.

In simple, plain English style, the book will guide you through the entire subject – the theories underlying hypnosis, the disorders it can be used to treat and the wide range of procedures and protocols for treating different conditions. You will find step-by-step guidance on how to conduct a course of therapy, from the initial consultation through establishing rapport with the client, taking a case history, deciding the appropriate techniques to use, setting realistic therapy aims and objectives, psycho-education, gathering of therapy resources, induction, deepening, therapeutic intervention, ego strengthening right through to bringing your client out of the trance. There is even a chapter that deals with all aspects of managing a successful therapy practice.

The book is aimed at practitioners and trainers, but it will also be of interest to psychology students, counsellors and anyone who is interested in the mind and personal growth.

Dr. Peter Marshall, BA., BSc., Ph.D., DCHyp., BST.Dip., is a distinguished psychologist whose books are sold worldwide in many different languages. He trained and qualified in hypnotherapy and psychotherapy at The Brief Strategic Therapy Foundation, London, and some of the scripts he was taught there are reproduced in this book. He is also a former examiner in psychology for a major Oxford and Cambridge examination board and the former Principal of the London School of Hypnotherapy and Psychotherapy.

1

What is Hypnosis?

The term hypnotherapy refers to two separate processes working together for a common purpose – hypnotism and therapy. The therapy involved in psychotherapy, is treatment to correct faults of the mind or mental processes. Hypnotism is an aid to carrying out this treatment successfully and quickly.

What hypnotherapists can treat

The mind problems that a hypnotherapist seeks to treat are clinical in their nature. This is a term used to refer to mind problems caused by external conditions – the individuals' past interactions with others and with their environment. Stress from workload, moving house, financial insecurity, or from relationship difficulties falls into this category and it can result in clinical depression and anxiety. Anxiety and neuroses can develop from general feelings of intolerability of living or working conditions. Phobias and destructive habits develop from inappropriate memory storage of events and so on[1].

These are all problems that arise from things outside of the body and they are all a hypnotherapist should attempt to deal with. If they are due to internal factors, such as physiological damage, chemical imbalance, abnormalities or retardation of the brain the hypnotherapist should leave them alone. Attempts to treat them with hypnotherapy could make things worse.

Clinical illnesses range from the mildest disorders, which cause only slight discomfort or inconvenience, to very server disorders that debilitate the sufferer. They develop because intolerable or traumatic circumstances, together with the mind's responses to them, are stored in inappropriate ways in the unconscious. Often troublesome storage in the unconscious has slipped in without full critical scrutiny and evaluation by the ego [2] (the conscious part of the mind). When it is recalled, it is likewise recalled in an uncritical way, as if it is a self-evident fact, even when the conscious mind knows it is not.

---

[1] Marshall 2012, Ch. 15.
[2] Marshall 2012b p.33.

Hypnotherapy techniques

Various techniques are used to deal with these inappropriate storages in different ways. Cognitive therapy would teach a client to consciously address the problem and try to compensate for the emotional responses with conscious, intelligent ones. Behaviourist psychologists would encourage clients to act as if the thoughts and feelings are not there. The quickest and most powerful method, though, would be to match, or overlay the inappropriate storage with counteracting appropriate storage, implanted, undiluted and unmodified, just like the inappropriate storage that is causing the problem. To do this, however, you would have to get past the radar of the ego altogether, otherwise it would get scrutinised, evaluated and modified. That is where the hypnotism comes in. Before we get onto that subject, though, since the therapy involved will act on the unconscious mind we need to have a look at what this is and how it functions.

2

The Conscious and Unconscious Minds

The mind is split into two main parts – the unconscious and the conscious. We will deal with the latter first, as this is the fundament from which the other part derives.

The Unconscious

The unconscious is the fundamental part of the mind. It automatically controls the functions and actions of the individual, just as a computer does in a complex machine or a modern car engine. It is a reservoir of feelings, urges and repressed memories of anxiety, conflict and pain.

The two subdivisions of the unconscious

A distinction can be made between the personal unconsciousness and the non-personal unconscious. The former contains things like bodily processes and hereditary, physical information. It is because these processes are in the unconscious part of the mind that we are not aware of them. Nor are we aware of how our genes and biological drives are influencing our bodies and our behaviour; we just naturally follow the urges to behave in the ways that we do.

The non-personal unconscious

The non-personal unconscious also contains reflexes and instinctual behavioural forms, collectively known as our phylogenetic heritage. It contains symbols, mythical images, archetypes, and it also contains information relating to the process of holding back the mind's as yet unfolded potential. This reservoir known as entelechy contains both those potentials that are ready to mature (ripe entelechy) and those that are being held back (blocked entelechy). Archetypal information falls into this entelechy category in so far as individuals are genetically predisposed to perceive themselves and others through inborn archetypes.

The personal unconscious

The personal unconscious also contains unconscious memories. A typical example is the birth trauma. Any intolerably unpleasant experience may be buried into the unconscious by the repression process, in order to protect the ego from being overwhelmed by anxiety and pain.

The Power of the Unconscious

The unconscious mind is non-linear and non-structured in its organisation. The lack of such constraints makes it a terrain that can be traversed rapidly and directly, just as a random access memory of a computer can function much more quickly than a sequential processor. There is, therefore, potential for solutions to problems to present themselves much more quickly than solely through use of the conscious mind.

You can't access and navigate this terrain with your conscious mind, though. It will simply present you with the answers if it chooses to. Have you ever woken up with the answer to a problem you had been struggling with the previous day? That's an example of how the unconscious delivers its wisdom to the conscious. This could also partly explain why we remember things more easily when we relax, although the reduction of anxiety that obscures recall also plays a part.

The role of the unconscious in skills and rehearsed routines

Your unconscious mind can control your body to perform well-rehearsed routines and skills at least partly automatically[3]. An example is when you slip into "automatic pilot" while driving your car, when your mind becomes abstracted and thinks about things other than the road conditions.

Physical Superstrength

The power of the unconscious to influence the body has also been demonstrated by various documented cases of people who have accessed extraordinary physical strength resources when their survival, or that of a loved one, has been at risk.

The Conscious Mind

The conscious mind is that part of the mind that has been trained to look outwards on the world and back on itself. Its function is to attempt to make as much sense as it can of all the data that it perceives from the external world and from the influences it is receiving from within. It engages directly with the environment and develops intelligent theories, skills and protocols designed to maximise the welfare of the individual. It contains all we are currently aware of and a sub-section which contains memories that can be recalled at will.

---

[3] Marshall (2012) p.21.

The conscious mind stores data and information on the environment in which we live. It consistently attempts to match perceptual data and perceptual records of the past, forming perceptual hypotheses[4]. All this data is synthesised and used to guide various kinds of mental and physical activity.

The boundary between the conscious and the unconscious
When an individual identifies fully with the conscious part of their mind, everything outside the object of their perception recedes into the unconscious.

The conscious mind knows that there is a huge amount of information and data outside its present focus and much of which is actually outside of its perceptual reach. The boundary between the conscious and the unconscious is the point beyond which the perceptual processes cannot pick up the stored impressions, or has no concepts for them. That does not mean that no data from beyond that boundary will be processed. The unconscious processes all sensory data it receives, stores it, activates other storage to help it make sense of it, generates hypotheses, and it influences our behaviours on the basis of it.

Thresholds and what can cross them
The boundary is also known as the verge. Some kinds of data in the unconscious can cross into the conscious and the part where this can occur is known as a threshold. Other kinds of data cannot cross the verge in conscious perceptible form, but they have their effect on the conscious nevertheless. Examples are urges, inhibitions, unconscious preferences and the kinds of information that lie behind these in the unconscious, including things like archetypes and instincts.

Another threshold is the limits of the imagination - the availability of images, which is what the imagination consists of. These include symbols, patterns, shapes, models, archetypes and myths held in the sub-conscious mind and available to the consciousness. They are tools with which to perceive things.

Another boundary between the conscious and the unconscious is the part of the ego that performs a guardian role, preventing access by the consciousness to data or information that would threaten its stability or identity. This guardian part of the consciousness starts to develop in the pre-verbal stages of infancy.

---

[4] Marshall (2012) p.32.

Repression

It is this part of the mind, operating at the verge between the unconscious and the conscious, that carries out the process of repression[5,6,7], when conscious experience threatens to undermine the identity or traumatise the emotions. These memories are buried deeply out of reach, so that there is no marker there for the conscious mind to access them. Some, however, while they may be out of reach to normal consciousness, may be able to be consciously recalled under hypnosis. More will be said about this later in this chapter.

Mutually Protecting Parts

The conscious mind protecting the unconscious

The conscious mind has developed, through conscious learning, to protect the welfare of the individual, by direct interaction with the world of modern complexity, the like of which the unconscious could not deal. The reason it could not is that these new conditions have developed more quickly than the evolution of the species could keep up with. Part of the process involves protecting the unconscious mind, itself, from threats to its stability.

The unconscious mind protecting the conscious

Blocking refers to the unconscious mind blocking a natural potential from emerging, because it perceives it as a threat to the ego. An example might be a highly intelligent child that underachieves because he or she does not know how intelligent they are and are afraid of the insights that they appear to have, which may be different to those of their peers[8].

The pre-conscious

The pre-conscious is a part of the mind that contains memories that can be recalled at will. It also contains those that can't, as long as the reason they can't are of a non-neurotic kind of forgetting. By this, I mean that they have not been buried in the unconscious by a repression process.

How the unconscious learns

The unconscious has its own abilities to learn, but it learns in a different way to the conscious mind. It learns automatically, without the use of the will, by association, repetition and emotion.

---

[5] Marshall (2012) pp.150-151.

[6] Marshall (2012b) pp.50-51.

[7] Marshall (2012c) p.65.

[8] Marshall (2012d).

Deliver To:

Claire Jack

1 SHERWOOD ROAD

Rarewaves.com Ltd
Columbia House, Apollo Rise
Southwood,Farnborough
GU14 0GT,United Kingdom
sales@rarewaves.com
www.rarewaves.com

PRESTWICK

KA9 1EY

Order No:205-3797043-355 6317

Qty	Description	Price
	MARSHALL, PETER DR HANDBOOK OF HYPNOTHERA 8.70 : A	

Multiple orders may be sent seperately.
Shipping costs may be seperately invoiced.
Vat No: 86415481

Sub Total:	8.70
Shipping :	0.99
Total :	9.69

Order Num:205-3797043-355631 Marketplace:Amazon UK

Reason For Return (Please complete so we can process your return)

[ ]Damaged/Defective/Faulty [ ]Incorrect Item Received
[ ]Unwanted/Changed Mind   [ ]Other Reason (State)

Do you require a Replacement/Refund/Exchange?

[ ]Replacement
[ ]Refund
[ ]Exchange(Different Item) 15888050

For further information on our returns policies
please refer to the website where you placed
your order or contact our customer service
team on returns@rarewaves.com.

Learning by repetition

If the individual repeats an action over and over again, the unconscious will learn to influence its behaviour to make it continue to do so. The more the same information is stored the more the memory trace is written in the same areas of the brain. The more it is overwritten the bolder the memory trace will be and just like a boldly written note is more likely to be seen than a faintly written one, so a boldly written memory trace is more likely to be recalled than a faintly written one. The stronger the trace becomes the more likely that it will influence the body or the mind, either through unconsciously controlling the body function, or by encouraging, or inhibiting mental activity.

Such actions will become habit. If a particular course of action makes an individual feel good the unconscious will encourage the repetition of that behaviour. In contrast, if an action makes the individual feel bad it will inhibit it.

Learning by association

Since the unconscious doesn't use logic, which is a learned, linear process, it can often be quicker than the conscious in finding a solution to a problem, because of its direct associative method. This is why solutions to problems can sometimes just spring into your head, as if from nowhere, like the warning messages that pop onto the screen of a computer, to warn you to do or not to do something.

The unconscious learns by association, for example, the smell of food will make you hungry, because it has stored these paired experiences so many times. When people hear jokes, jokes of their own spring to mind, because these behaviours (hearing and recalling jokes to tell) have been stored in pairs so many times before.

The purpose of the unconscious mind is to maximise the welfare of the individual, which includes keeping them safe from bodily and emotional harm. When a conscious experience occurs the unconscious compares it with similar experiences stored in the episodic memory.[9]

If these have been stored in association with reward, or a positive feeling, similar emotions will be felt. If, however, the previous experience was stored in association with a negative feeling, perhaps from a reprimand, a rejection, or a feeling of failure or inadequacy, this negative feeling will be recalled and will inhibit the individual from continuing or welcoming
the experience[10].

---

[9] Marshall (2012b) Ch.29.
[10] Marshall (2012 Ch.s 4 & 15.

Evaluations modify the associations

What will also be stored, however, if the person is consciously attending to the experience, or data input, will be an evaluation and judgement of it by the consciousness. Therefore, input of things we are told, shown, or that we consciously attend to enter the episodic and other memory centres in qualified form.

The way memory recall happens, whether it is recalled into the consciousness or the unconsciousness, is the same way as the data went in. Therefore, if something we are told is judged by our ego with reservations, perhaps that it is only probably, or even possibly correct, or valid, or significant, perhaps that it is only partially correct, or perhaps that it applies in most, some, or only few instances, it will be recalled as such. Nothing that the ego intercepts goes in unqualified, or taken for granted.

No long-term strategist

The unconscious is no long-term strategist though; it cannot work out what the long-term consequences of any behaviour will be, or put together a plan of combined actions to bring about a desired goal. It has no judgemental ability. It just learns everything that it encounters - bad habits as well as good. Only the learned, intelligent, conscious part of the mind can make judgements.

The unconscious mind will simply give you more of what you have already had in terms of thoughts and behaviour.

The unconscious influences our body and behaviour

Psychoanalytical theory provides that our behaviour is driven by inner, unconscious forces of which we are unaware. It is now well established that the biological functioning of the body is also influenced by the mind.

Every idea, emotion, thought and belief gives rise to neurochemical messages through the central nervous system. The messengers are long-chain molecules known as neuropeptides. These molecules and their receptors are also found in the brain and the immune system, indicating that all these parts are involved in the common communication network. The chemical messages influence our emotions and our physiology and these, in turn, feedback to our unconscious mind and sometimes also to our conscious mind, in terms of sensations.

Conscious unawareness of the unconscious

We are not consciously aware of how the brain and mind move and change the state of our bodies, for example when we go from wakefulness to sleep. Nor are we aware of the process by which the unconscious keeps out of the reach of our consciousness.

It could be that its threshold is kept at bay by fear that we would be overwhelmed by its contents if we could access them. It could be a conscious choice not to be aware of everything we are doing. Think of what happens when you become aware of your breathing. Many people find they become uncomfortable; they may yawn repeatedly or may get out of breath. Think, also, of what happens when you become aware that you are making eye contact during a conversation. It is much more comfortable when you are unaware that you are doing so.

It is reasonable to assume that we keep the unconscious out of reach by inattention to it because:

- we are busy attending to other things
- we have no appropriate concepts through which to perceive it
- of anxiety experienced when we get near the perceptual threshold
- of the absorbing nature of interaction with the external world.

Fast working
These neurochemicals work fast and the effects are relatively long lasting. A fear stimulus will make your body react with fight or flight symptoms very quickly, but it will take a longer time for the feelings to subside after the threat has gone. Likewise, if something makes you feel happy or sad, the emotion will persist

The unconscious mind and physical health
Because of this close association between our unconscious mind and our bodily functions, the workings of the unconscious mind are closely related to our physical health, as well as our mental health.

If a person is feeling depressed the body will interpret their emotion and produce a state of lethargy in their body movement. It's because their unconscious tends to assist them to do what it thinks they want to do.

The well established, placebo effect, where tablets that contain nothing but sugar have an efficacious effect on illness, is an example of how the mind influences the functioning and the health of the body.

Stress and physical illness
It is well known that stress – a mental phenomenon, since it is the perception of inability to cope – causes, through unconscious processes, heart disease, stomach ulcers and weakening of the immune system.

Discovery of the fight or flight response mechanism

In the early part of the twentieth century, Walter Cannon[11] discovered that human beings have a built in *fight or flight response mechanism.* It is the name he gave to the way our unconscious mind responds to perceived threats.

When something frightens us our body goes into fight or flight response mode. The unconscious mind, misunderstanding the real, modern-day nature of the threat, prepares it for a physical act of defence or an escape run. It does this by triggering the secretion of hormones that alter the balance of physiological systems in the body, particularly the thyroid, the adrenal glands and the pituitary. Blood is sent rushing to our muscles to provide extra strength. Our heart rate increases. Our blood vessels narrow in the process and this causes an inevitable increase in our blood pressure. Our Urinary and diuretic processes are stimulated, in order to lighten the weight of the body for a faster getaway. Hunger is suppressed, our immune system is alerted and the stress hormones: cortisone, cortisol and corticosteroid are produced and sent around our bloodstream ready to mend injury damage.

The maladaptive nature of the response

The fight or flight response is almost always at error. It has been shaped by evolutionary forces over millions of years, during most of which the only kinds of threats to the individual were physical ones, threats of death or injury by another of the species or a predatory animal. There is no one to fight and nowhere to run to where most modern threats are concerned, though, for example, the threat of losing one's job, or not being able to pay the bills. Since evolution takes a long time and humans have been civilised for only a tiny fraction of the evolutionary journey it is not surprising that this biological structure has not caught up with the changing conditions of life.

The adrenaline that is generated to pump blood to the muscles therefore goes to waste. The stress chemicals that are generated to mend injury are not needed and this situation causes physiological damage of its own. The extra gastric acid that is produced just causes stomach ulcers and continued raised blood pressure makes the individual susceptible to heart disease.

Soon after Cannons' discovery, Seyle[12] discovered that if this disturbance continues for a prolonged period of time it leads to a shrinking of the thymus and other organs. This has important

---

[11] Cannon (1929)
[12] Seyle (1955)

consequences for the health of an individual. The immune system works by producing antibodies to fight off disease organisms in the bloodstream, but these antibodies themselves can become so numerous that that the surplus begins to attack the healthy parts of the individual. The various forms the damage can take are known as autoimmune diseases and include things like cancer and AIDS.

To protect against this happening, lymphocytes are produced in bone marrow. These are known as B cells. Some of these migrate to the thymus where they multiply and become what are known as Killer T Cells. These patrol the bloodstream and attack any cells that have become mutated or abnormal. When the thymus shrinks the body's ability to produce these killer T Cells diminishes and therefore leaves the body under-defended against such autoimmune diseases.

Neuro-immunology
By the time of Seyle's discovery, the integral nature of the mind-body system was well established. It was known that every emotion, thought, belief, or idea that occurred in the mind has a physiological consequence.

There is now a whole academic discipline under the name of neuro-immunology, the focus of which is bi-directional communication between the nervous, endocrine and the immune systems and the relationship between this and human health. This is providing us with an increasing understanding of the ways the mind influences the body to help it combat disease. The dominant figure in this field to date has been Ernest Rossi.

Research in this field has demonstrated that people's thoughts and emotions can generate good health. Robert Ader[13], working in the field of psycho-neuro-immunology, believes this strong link between our minds and our bodies can enable us to heal our own ills.

Importance of expressing emotions
Studies in neuro-immunology have shown the importance of expressing emotions appropriately. When strong feelings of fear, anger, or rage are not expressed fully and appropriately, the inappropriate feelings are stored. This produces an excess of epinephrine, which, in turn, causes chemical breakdown, weakening the immune system and rendering the individual susceptible to disease. It is, therefore, important to express emotions and not block them verbally or physically.

---

[13] Ader (2007)

Other errors of the unconscious
The unconscious also makes errors in the way it learns from experience. It doesn't have the faculty of judgment. Therefore, it will learn bad habits just as well as it will learn good ones, because it simply learns by repetition and association[14]. If you repeat an action, it will learn it and influence you to go on repeating it. If an action gives you short-term pleasure (or relief from anxiety, which is essentially the same thing) it will learn it, and predispose you to repeat it, even if it does you harm in the long term. This is because it is the quick reward that it registers. Fifteen to thirty seconds afterward is the optimum time for the effectiveness of a reward[15].

When a smoker is stressed and lights up a cigarette the chemicals in the smoke, together with the distraction that that the action gives them, will relieve their negative feelings in the short term. In consequence, the act of smoking will be stored in association with relief from anxiety. When the person feels stressed again they will recall, either consciously or unconsciously, the relief the cigarette gave them and will desire a cigarette again. The long –term consequences, however, are that smoking will damage their health and make them less able to cope with stress. Moreover, they will eventually experience new stress from smoking related disease.

Practicing imperfectly
Another way the unconscious makes errors is by practicing imperfectly. Practice makes perfect, but only if you practice the best possible technique; otherwise you become very good at doing something baldly[16].

Errors that cause neurosis
The unconscious makes errors in its learning in ways that inappropriately influence mental life too. Phobias are an example. One of the main ways that phobias develop is when a fear feeling is experienced consciously, for some normal, fear-provoking reason (e.g. a loud noise) while the image of something else (e.g. a spider) is perceived in the peripheral vision. The latter perception is, therefore, subliminal and, therefore, escapes the scrutiny of the ego. As a result, an association between the image of a spider and a feeling of anxiety is stored, uncritically.

If the ego had been aware of the spider it would have noted that it had nothing to do with the loud and frightening noise. The association

---

[14] Marshall (2012e) p.21)
[15] Marshall (2012b) p.31.
[16] Marshall (2012e), p.21.

would still have been stored but it would have been stored with the qualification that the two were causally unconnected.

Superstitions

Superstitions are another kind of storage error that the unconscious mind makes. Their common kinds probably originated in the same way as other maladaptations. Inevitably, there will have been people who experienced a negative event following a time when a single Magpie was in their vision. Their unconscious mind will have stored the temporal association. In many cases, the association may have even been made consciously with the same irrationally perceived meaning, thus, reinforcing the erroneous storage in the unconscious mind.

Many of the superstitions that are around today date back to times when the thinking of common people was less rational than it is today and magical ideas were more prevalent. The world was a more mysterious place and people resorted to occult explanations in the absence of scientific understanding. These superstitions, therefore, spread from person to person.

Whichever is the main process by which superstitious associations originated the mechanism by which they become established, persistent and influential in the mind of an individual is the same. It is a matter of a different kind of well-meaning mischief from the unconscious mind. The latter seeks to maintain the stability of the ego and senses, rightly or wrongly, at times that harsh reality is more than it can take. It therefore encourages the ego to shift its focus away from reality towards an irrational problem with which it assumes it can more easily cope, particularly if it has done so many times before. These irrational associations, learnt from others, provide ready distractions for it to use in this way.

Defence mechanisms

Defence mechanisms are processes through which the unconscious shields the conscious mind from the reality of a particular fact or circumstance[17,18]. Here it is the conscious ego that drives the process, putting things out of reach by burying them in the unconscious.

In some cases, such protection may be useful, but psychotherapists would argue that such mechanisms lie at the root of neuroses and are, therefore, maladaptations.

---

[17] Marshall (2012) p.150-151.
[18] Marshall (2012b) p.44-51.

Examples are:

- Projection
- Denial
- Displacement
- Reaction formation
- Rationalisation
- Regression

All involve repression, i.e. burying some data or information in the unconscious. These devices are ways of concealing that something has been repressed.

Projection
Projection is where the conscious mind buries guilt in the unconscious and distracts the individual's attention from the hiding place by pointing the finger at someone else.

Denial
Denial is where a fact that causes too much anxiety for the ego to cope with is buried in the unconscious and attention is kept away from it by denial that it ever was a valid truth.

Displacement
Displacement is a process whereby a fact or set of circumstances, too painful or anxiety provoking to deal with, is buried in the unconscious and the emotional response directed, instead, towards another, more manageable problem.

Reaction Formation
A reaction formation is where an intolerable awareness of something is buried in the unconscious and covered up by acting as if the very opposite were the case.

Rationalisation
Rationalisation is a way that an ego may sometimes deal with a set of circumstances which it cannot tolerate. It buries the intolerable essence of the situation in the unconscious and conceals it with a cognitive restructuring, or reconceptualisation of the issue, to make it acceptable. Guilt feelings are sometimes dealt with in this way

Regression

Regression is a process where, to escape an intolerable situation, or fact, an individual regresses, mentally, to a time before which the intolerable situation or fact existed. The offending fact and the situation in which it occurred are then out of reach of the consciousness; they exist only in the unconscious.

Conscious control of the unconscious

So we've established that the unconscious influences the conscious, but is there any defensible reason to think that the latter also has any influence on the former? This would be necessary if conscious correction of its faults is to be achieved. Well, the defence mechanisms above are manifestations of such a direction of influence. There are also various, well-established channels of influence that bridge the boundary between the conscious and the unconscious. Here is a list of examples:

- The immune system
- Breathing
- Imagery
- Emotions
- Colours
- Pain

The immune system

It has been well established that the immune system of the body is heavily influenced by the unconscious mind and this is something we can see directly. It has been demonstrated by Robert Ader[19], at the University of Rochester, New York, that the immune system in mice can be conditioned. This then suggests that the unconscious mind can be conditioned consciously, at least by a therapist. To the extent that the therapist is acting on the conscious instructions of the client, it follows that the client is consciously influencing their unconscious, even if indirectly so.

Breathing bridges the boundary

Breathing is a process that is partly unconscious and partly conscious. Therefore, it forms a bridge between the two states. Most of the time we breathe without being aware of it, but we can focus upon it and we can also control it consciously.

Because it has one foot in the conscious world, we can use this to control what is a partly unconscious process and therefore, to some

---

[19] Ader (2007)

degree, control the unconscious itself. For example, when we feel stressed and our unconscious mind has activated the fight or flight response, sending the hormonal system into overdrive, we tend to breathe fast and shallowly. We can, however, consciously control that breathing which manifests its behaviour in the conscious mind, and make it slow and deep instead. This then influences what is going on in the unconscious, as its other foot, so to speak, is planted there. It forces that part of the mind to act as though the threat is not so great. This, in turn, causes the parasympathetic nervous system to direct the adrenal system and other parts of the process of preparation for fight or flight to stand down.

Biofeedback systems demonstrate the 2-way process
Biofeedback systems demonstrate that conscious control of the unconscious is possible. These are electronic machines that monitor muscle relaxation, heart rate, breathing and perspiration. The live data is available to the individual, who can then consciously reduce the excitement of their autonomic nervous system by breathing control, visualisation of imagery and muscle relaxation.

Guided imagery
Imagination guided by a therapist has been well established to reduce stress. It increases the positiveness of the client's outlook and this increased optimism boosts their immune system, which is, itself, governed by the unconscious.

Emotions
The most powerful driver of all where the unconscious mind is concerned is emotion and words have a very powerful effect on the latter. Emotion is what primarily drives motivation and outlook.

Colours influence the unconscious
Some authorities have argued that colours have an influence on the unconscious. This would seem reasonable.

Green is likely to be associated, in the unconscious, with a state of well-being, as it is the colour that has probably become ingrained as natural in the genetics of our memory system. It would seem reasonable to assume that over many generations, most of which would have been in forest rather than urban environments, the human race would have become naturally selected to favour this colour. It will have been the most conducive to survival, much more so than blue, which would be suggestive of open space, where the sky can be seen. It would have been in such spaces that our early ancestors would have been highly vulnerable. It is also suggestive of the sea, where they could easily drown.

Likewise, favouring yellow would not have been conducive to survival, as it would suggest favouring dry and barren deserts.

Pain and the unconscious

Another way that the unconscious communicates with the conscious mind is through pain. Conversely the conscious can control the unconscious and, in turn, the body, by conscious control of this pain, whether by drugs or by other means, such as hypnosis.

NLP

Neuro-linguistic programming theory provides that there is a physiological counterpart to any state of mind. If we can recognise this counterpart we can use it as a handle to control our states of mind[20].

While the states of mind are experienced consciously the physiological counterpart is produced unconsciously. We would not normally consciously decide to smile when we feel happy or consciously decide to hold our head in our hands when we feel worried or sad. We just do these things automatically, driven by the unconscious.

Neuro-linguistic programming utilises this connection. The theory provides that if we consciously perform the physiological counterpart the desired state of mind will materialise[21].

Consciously correcting storage errors in the unconscious

Can we use our conscious mind, with its intelligent, analytical and judgmental abilities, to correct the storage errors our unconscious mind makes? Well we can if we can get past the guard's attention. The guard is the ego, which scrutinises and evaluates everything that enters our perception, thereby modifying the way it is subsequently stored.

There was a time in everyone's life when powerful suggestions could be implanted without inducing a special state of consciousness. The ego that scrutinises and evaluates input is not fully developed before the age of about five. Without a mature ego, the infant child just takes in what it is told and accepts it, uncritically, as fact.

If it goes in as a self-evident truth, needing no justification, it will come out in the same way. This is why values implanted early stick throughout life. This is why behavioural inhibitions and beliefs persist

---

[20] Marshall (2012c).
[21] Marshall (2012c) Ch. 4.

into adulthood even if the conscious mind tells the beholder that they are unjustified and inappropriate in the modern age. It explains, for example, prejudices.

Correcting the Errors

If only we could recreate those conditions for data input that existed before the individual was out of infancy, before the ego was fully developed. Well, obviously, we can't turn back the clock but we can do the next best thing. There are ways in which we can catch the ego unawares and so implant counteracting data without it knowing. We can then influence the individual with a similarly permanent effect as the parent of an infant child does. This data will be stored without modification or qualification, just as the data that is causing a problem may have entered. How can we do it? We can do it by creating a hypnoidal state.

Hypnoidal States

There are times when the conscious mind has almost gone to sleep and you can sneak suggestions in without it noticing. These are hypnoidal states. Some of them occur naturally. Examples are:

- Hypnopompic states
- Hypnogogic states
- Daydreaming

Hypnopompic states

A hypnopompic state is that state when your conscious mind is beginning to switch off, when you are between waking and sleeping. Bizarre experiences can occur because your conscious, rational mind is beginning to switch off and it is your unconscious, the part that is not rational, that is becoming dominant. It's one of those times when you are highly likely to give nonsensical answers to things people say and, when challenged, you will suddenly respond with something like "Oh. I was nearly asleep." Only your conscious mind can deliver intelligent communications to others and it was not awake.

Hypnogogic states

Hypnogogic states are the similar states that occur when you are just waking up in the morning.

Daydreaming states

Daydreaming is yet another example, when you seem to be miles away from what is going on in front of you. The guard of consciousness - the sentry to the unconscious part of your mind has almost gone to sleep.

Hypnotists use hypnoidal states
Each of these states involves physical and mental relaxation and some degree of detachment from the immediate, real world. They exist at the margin between consciousness and unconsciousness and it is here where suggestions can be made to the unconscious without scrutiny of the consciousness. Hypnotists can deliberately induce such states.

How a hypnotherapist can induce a hypnoidal state
A hypnotherapist can induce a hypnoidal state by:

- Deep relaxation techniques, or
- Overloading the consciousness by distraction or confusion.

Why suggestions implanted in this way are so powerful
The unconscious accepts the suggestions uncritically, because they have not been run past the judgement of the consciousness, and the unconscious does not have any judgment of its own. Furthermore, since episodic memory traces are only laid down as a result of consciously processing information, the individual will have no recollection of the suggestions implanted. The suggestions will affect their behaviour thereafter in the same powerful way as those of parents of infant children will affect their behaviour even in adulthood.

Induced hypnoidal states are essentially similar to the naturally occurring hypnoidal states and are nothing for anyone to be afraid of. Just like the naturally occurring ones, a person can snap out of them whenever they chose. If they should drift off to sleep they will no longer be in a hypnoidal state, but in a normal sleep state and this is natural and essential to us all. No therapist can influence a client in that state.

The following chapters will guide you on how to bring about the deep relaxation state required for this, the ways of overloading the consciousness if that option is selected, the forms of suggestion to make for particular purposes, the manner of implanting them and then how to bring your client gently out of the hypnotic state.

3

A Brief History of Hypnosis

Hypnosis in ancient times

Hypnosis has a long history. It hasn't always been called hypnosis, but the technique has been used since time immemorial.

Ancient witchdoctors used rituals, rhythmic drumbeats, dances and psychoactive drugs to induce trance states and cure maladies. Kroger and Fezler[22] report that the ancient Hebrews used magical rites, incantation, meditation, breathing exercises and fixation on Hebrew letters of the alphabet.

The essence of what we now call hypnotherapy was practiced by the ancient Hindus and Sikhs in India. The latter had sleep temples for the purpose, as did ancient Greece and Egypt. Egyptian, archaeological records refer to the incubation or sleep temples of Imhotep, the first known physician, and the ancient Greeks had shrines of healing, where patients would receive suggestions while in an induced sleep.

The first written record

The Persian psychologist and physician Avicenna wrote about the practice in The *Book of Healing,* in 1027 AD.

Hypnosis in the first millennium

Franz Anton Mesmer

Centuries later, Franz Anton Mesmer, a medical student in the late 18th century, discovered that he could cure a person's malady by passing magnets over their body. He later found that he could achieve the same effect merely with his hands and eyes and inferred that these were sources of a kind of animal magnetism. He argued that this process could unblock the flow of this magnetism in the bodies of his patients, thereby relieving the illnesses which such blockage was causing.

---

[22] (1976)

It was this that first made the subject well known in the West. The animal magnetism theory was later to be debunked, but hypnotism is still, today, often referred to as mesmerism.

The Marquis de Puysegur

Mesmer's student, The Marquis de Puysegur, found he could induce sleep in his patients and still converse with them, but that they would not remember the experience after he brought them out of the sleep. Puysegur believed that the will of the patient was important in the process.

Abbe Faria

In Paris, in the early part of the 19th century, a Roman Catholic monk named Abbe Faria introduced a version of the technique. Faria understood that it was not due to any special power emanating from the hypnotist, but that it was due to the power of suggestion in the mind of the patient. His method of induction into a hypnotic state was by command following expectancy.

James Braid

It was a 19th century Scottish surgeon called James braid who coined the terms *hypnosis* and *hypnotism*. He found that the trance could be induced by focusing on a bright object such as his silver watch. Once induced and brought out of the trance of patient could be induced quickly by a single word.

He argued that this state was induced by prolonged ocular fixation fatiguing certain areas of the brain, resulting in a sleep of the nerves. The Greek language, which has traditionally been a predominant source of medical terminology, contained terms for this *hypnos*, the god of sleep and *neuro*, for nerves. From this, Braid coined the term *neuro-hypnotism*. As time went by the *neuro* prefix was dropped. Unfortunately this, together with the earlier sleep temples that were used in ancient times, has led to the enduring error in people's minds that hypnotism has anything to do with sleep in the conventional sense of the word. The term *hypnosis* is, therefore, a misnomer.

The first book on hypnosis

It was Braid who published the first known book on hypnosis – *Neurypnology (1843)* and he is regarded by many as the founder of modern hypnosis and hypnotherapy.

John Ellison

The technique was not readily accepted by everyone. In fact, John Ellison (1791 -- 1868), professor of medicine at UCL was disbarred from his profession for demonstrating the technique.

James Esdaile
The first record of hypnosis being used as an anaesthetic in surgical operation in the relatively modern world was in the mid-19th century, by surgeon James Esdaile (1808 - 1859). It may have been used before, as far back as ancient times, for it is known from archaeological finds that primitive operations were carried out, but we have no actual record to support the use of hypnosis as an anaesthetic in them.

Ambriose-Auguste Liebeault and The Nancy School
In 1866, The Nancy School in Paris became the dominant centre for hypnosis and there, its founder, Ambriose-Auguste Liebeault, a disciple of Faria (see p.32) established the crucial importance of co-operation between hypnotists and their subjects. Liebeault is also regarded by many as the father of modern hypnotherapy.

Hyppolyte Bernheim
In about 1880, Hyppolyte Bernheim joined the Nancy School and became influential in the research and development of the practice. He discovered that some subjects were more suggestible than others were, but he was criticised for failing to recognise the importance of rapport between the hypnotist and their patient.

Albert Moll and Boris Sidis
From the Nancy School, modern interest in the subject of hypnotherapy spread to other parts of the world, through, attendees such as Albert Moll to the United States of America and Boris Sidis and Morton Prince to Germany.

Sidis defined the concept of suggestibility as follows:

> "Suggestibility varies as the amount of disaggression and inversely as the unification of consciousness. Disaggression refers to the split between the normal waking consciousness and the sub consciousness. "

Acceptability was growing
The practice was becoming more acceptable by this time. Some in the Church were dubious about it, but others accepted it. It was employed in the treatment of injured soldiers in the American Civil War.

In 1889, Paris held the first International Congress on hypnosis and in 1892, its use was unanimously endorsed by the BMA in Britain.

Jean-Martin Charcot and the Paris School

Jean-Martin Charcot is a name that tends to be prominently associated with hypnotism during the second half of the 19th century, particularly because Sigmund Freud was a student of his. However, Charcot's contribution to the theory was actually little and he promulgated the erroneous conception that if a person was found to be hypnotically suggestible that was an indication that they were mentally ill.

He deduced that a trance was a kind of seizure because it appeared to be similar to epilepsy symptoms. He also believed that hysteria, the mental illness to which he was referring, was due to hereditary neurological faults.

Later, however, he did accept that psychologically healthy people could also be hypnotically suggestible. Where this was the case, he referred to it as petite hypnotisme, in contrast to the pathological kind, which he termed grande hypnotisme.

Public demonstrations

Charcot was well known for his public demonstrations of hypnosis, yet, ironically, he argued that the sensationalism surrounding the practice damaged its research value.

Hypnosis in the 20th century

Emile Coué

At the beginning of the 20th century, Emile Coué joined the Nancy school and developed a version of hypnotherapy which he called autosuggestion. The basic principle was his discovery of the placebo effect on illness and his inference from that, that if a person repeated words suggesting improvement in their malady enough, their unconscious mind would accept them and they would have their own placebo effect.

Breuer

Freud's associate, Breuer, used hypnosis to induce a catharsis, or emotional outpouring of past events and found that the patients' symptoms disappeared as a result. Freud, however, found he could achieve the same result (an abreaction) without the use of hypnosis.

Use of hypnosis for treating battle trauma

The two world wars, plus the Korean War saw hypnosis again being used for battle trauma, particularly in treating battle neurosis.

Schultz
The German surgeon, Schultz, developed a method that he called autogenic training to treat trauma in soldiers in the last world war.

Hilgard and Muller/The Stanford laboratory
From then on, the scientific study of hypnosis became more serious. The Stanford laboratory of hypnosis research was founded in 1957 and there, Ernest Hilgard and Andre Muller Weitzenhoffer produced the Stanford hypnotic suggestibility scales.

Neodissociation theory
Hilgard established what is known as the neodissociation theory of hypnotism. This provides that a person undergoing hypnosis can be aware of pain without feeling the discomfort.

Some critics argued that this was merely a consequence of the instructions given during the hypnosis session. Hildegard, however, believed that we all have a second being sharing our consciousness, which we are unaware of, but which observes and warns us in some way if we are in danger - a kind of guardian angel.

This is an idea that has been around since times of antiquity. The two parts to the psyche are known to the chinese as the *hun* and the *po*. They were known to the ancient Egyptians as the *ka* and the *ba* and to the ancient Greeks as the *dæmon* and the *eidolon*.

The empirical basis of Hilgard's inference
Hilgard arrived at this conclusion after an experiment, where a blind person was hypnotised to become deaf. As a result, the person could not hear anything, not even loud sounds next to his ear. He could not even hear any further suggestions or commands from the hypnotist.

Hilgard then spoke quietly to his ear and suggested that there may be some part of him that could hear his words. If so, he asked that that part to communicate it to him by raising the index finger. The index finger did raise and when the subject emerged from the trance he described his experience in the trance as being able to hear absolutely nothing, but that he had been aware of his index finger moving and was curious to know why it did so. He was not aware that the hypnotist had made the request. That, Hilgard inferred, must have been picked up by the hidden observer.

In another experiment, one of Hilgard's subjects referred to being aware of what seemed to be her *higher self,* acting relatively separately from her ego.

The hidden observer
The hidden observer, Hilgard believed, sees everything that is going on, like a guardian angel, but communicating it to the consciousness is usually unnecessary. The hidden observer is also what protects us from doing anything under hypnosis that we would not normally choose to do, such as cause harm to another person.

This, you will realise, as you read further on in this book, is the theoretical basis of the technique known as *parts therapy*.

Andrew Salter and conditioned reflex therapy.
Behavioural studies have since shown that certain physical capacities can be enhanced by use of hypnosis. In 1940, Andrew Salter combined it with Pavlovian conditioning to treat behavioural inhibitions that he believed were the underlying cause of most neuroses. His method is known as *conditioned reflex therapy*.

Regulation and recommendation
From there on the acceptance of hypnosis developed rapidly and so did its formal regulation. *The British hypnotism Act* was passed in 1952. Its use was approved by the BMA in 1955, for treatment of psychoneurosis and for anaesthesia in childbirth. It also recommended that doctors should receive training in the subject.

Milton Erickson
Milton Erickson has been the greatest influence on the development of modern hypnotherapy. His methods often departed from what had become the orthodoxy of practice. He didn't necessarily go through the usual protocol of inducing advance. He would, instead, endeavour to enter into the patient's world, using confirming statements, humour and surprise, evoking useful imagery and use of metaphor. As a result of this artful and insightful process the client would slide into a hypnotic trance.

4

The Pre- induction Interview

The objectives
There are four objectives of the pre-induction interview:

- Gathering information about the client, their problem and any therapy resources that can be utilised
- Eliciting their expectancy of cure
- Removing any fears or misconceptions he/she has about hypnosis
- Building rapport with the client

Making the appointment
When you speak to a client to make an appointment, be business-like rather than chatty. Listen attentively, but don't allow the caller to go on too long. The place for this is in your consulting room, not on the telephone. You only need enough information to decide whether you are likely to be able to help them. If so, invite them to make an appointment.

Mode of dress
When the client attends your consulting room image is important. It is advisable to dress in a business suit, or smart casuals. Some therapists dress rather Bohemian. A therapist I knew in the North of England routinely dressed in Bavarian style shorts and a straw hat with two tall feathers sticking out of the back of it. He had a small clientele who seemed to stay with him for years and who thought he was the best thing since sliced bread, but most non-clients tended to think he was slightly barmy. His fee income was never enough to keep him, for he had to resort to other part-time jobs to supplement it.

Its best, in my opinion, to go the whole hog and dress smart and business-like. Symbols of authority are very powerful in these situations and you need as much authority as you can achieve if you are to obtain the best results for your client. Dressing casually, or worse, dressing Bohemian, may make you feel good, but it is your client who is paying the bills; it's him or her that you are being paid to make feel good.

Personal hygiene
Personal hygiene is important. Body odour, dirty nails or clothing, unkempt, greasy hair obviously give the wrong impression, but overpowering perfume or aftershave can also be very off-putting.

The consulting room
The consulting room should be neutral and uncluttered. Magnolia, or cream paint is ideal. Have no religious, or political symbols or literature around
   The phones should be switched off, unless they are in another room and there is someone to answer them.

Be attentive
Be a patient listener. Display receptive body language and use pacing and mirroring of the client's behaviour appropriately. Speak clearly with good diction; even this is a symbol of authority that will enhance the trust the client has in you.

Confidentiality
Assure the client that everything they tell you will be treated in the strictest confidence

Professional distance
Spend a few minutes getting to know the client, but don't overdo it. You need to keep a professional distance, rather than becoming chummy. Ask them why they have come to see you, why they have chosen to try hypnotism to resolve, or relieve, their problem and what they hope to achieve through the treatment, in terms of degree of cure or relief.

Allaying fears and misconceptions
One of the objectives of pre-induction talk is to allay any fears or misconceptions the client has about hypnotherapy. Here are some of the most common:

- It may be a waste of money
- The therapist will override their own will
- They will make themselves vulnerable to sexual assault
- They may reveal secrets
- They will lose control
- They may get stuck in the trance

- They will be asleep and won't remember anything
- They may be left with a post hypnotic suggestion implanted that may be harmful to themselves or others

Reassuring your client

Assure your client of the following facts. With the kind of induction you will be using - deep relaxation - they will always be in control throughout the hypnosis session.

They should not believe what they see on television. What they see in hypnotism entertainment shows is not really hypnotism at all; it is more a case of selecting the most socially compliant characters, who will, however wittingly or unwittingly, subject themselves to the will of another. It is more compliance than anything else. The participants know what the role of a stage hypnotist's subject is and some people are highly role-compliant. It is this more than the power of the hypnotist that produces the effects in these shows.

The effects that are seen on the stage are due to a multiplicity of influences, most of which are nothing to do with hypnotism and to do justice to the analogy would require another book on its own. Suffice it to say here that professional hypnotherapy in the consulting room is nothing like these shows.

Your client has no cause to fear that they will be made to do anything they do not choose to do. They remain in control. If they were unconscious, or asleep, the therapy would not work, as their mind has to be listening. They will remain awake and aware of everything around them. They will be highly relaxed and receptive to suggestions, but their conscious mind will still be alert and ready to protect them if there is a threat. The unconscious mind is always alert, watching, and ready to override the conscious mind if and when it perceives a threat.

This is why people sometimes become frightened of something they know they should not really be scared of - a spider, for example. It's because their unconscious mind has the upper hand. Whatever their conscious, analytical mind is doing the unconscious has the power to override it if it feels it should do.

Everyone can be hypnotised

As to whether it will be a waste of money, clients who voice this concern generally mean that they may not be able to be hypnotised. If they say, straight out, that they cannot be hypnotised, agree with them. Tell them they can only hypnotise themselves, but the hypnotist can assist them as an expert facilitator.

Assure them that everyone can be guided into a trance. Tell them that as long as they do exactly as you say they will definitely become hypnotised. Explain that all hypnosis is self-hypnosis and you are an expert in guiding a person into this state of mind. The only one who can prevent them being hypnotised is they themselves if they really do not want to be.   When you do your suggestibility tests you can demonstrate your point. Suggestibility tests will be deal with shortly.

Fear that they may reveal secrets

With regard to a client's fear that they may reveal secrets that they don't want to reveal, explain that people are just as able and ready to lie under hypnosis as they are in everyday life. If they consciously don't want to reveal something in their normal everyday state of mind they won't reveal it under hypnosis. The unconscious mind performs a guardian role in relation to the conscious mind and is in overall control at all times. You will only do or say things while under hypnosis that you want to do or say. Nobody can make you do or say what you don't want to.

Fear of getting stuck in a trance

With regard to the fear of getting stuck in a trance permanently, reassure your client as follows. Getting stuck in a trance could never happen, as their conscious mind (their ego) is in overall control all of the time, just the same as when a trance state occurs when driving a car or watching the film. You can always remove yourself from that trance any time you want to, or need to. The reason the trance endures as long as it does is simply that you allow it to do so. It is the same with hypnosis. You will only stay in the trance as long as you want to. If you choose to remain in it, it will be because you find it comfortable, just as you might choose to remain in a daydream or reading a book.

The most that could happen is that you might fall asleep, just as when you get comfortable in front of the television. You will, in due course, wake up and think " Oh! I must have drifted off."   In fact, you are in a naturally occurring trance every night, just before you go to sleep and, again, just after you wake up. These are called hypnagogic and hypnopompic states. They are when you're in a half-waking state. In fact, you can use self-induced trance to send yourself to sleep at night. I do it all the time.

Concern that they will be asleep and not remember anything

Regarding any fear that they will be asleep and won't remember anything, explain that this is a misconception and that they will not actually be asleep at all in the usual sense of the word. Indeed, if they were the hypnotherapy wouldn't work. It will simply be a state of deep relaxation, where their conscious mind will be able to communicate with their unconscious in a way that is not available in everyday states of mind, because this connection is not available under normal circumstances

When you know, in your conscious mind, that your responses to certain stimuli have no basis in intelligence, reason or logic, but, in spite of this, they persist habitually, defying your reason, this is because the part of your mind that uses these validation criteria (the conscious mind) is normally not able to access and manipulate the part of your mind that doesn't (the unconscious mind). The hypnotic induction enables your consciousness to be in contact and communication with your unconscious and to make changes, so that the irrational impulses don't override the conscious mind any more.

Fear that they will be giving up control to the therapist

As to a client's concern that they will be giving up control to the therapist, explain that they won't. That's not the therapist's intention. The goal is for the therapist to put the two parts of their own mind into communication with each other, a state that does not normally exist, and the therapist will only be doing this by assisting them to self-hypnotise. In fact, all hypnosis is self-hypnosis. The hypnotist is just a guide and facilitator.

Fear of being left with a harmful post-hypnotic suggestion implanted

As for the fear that they may be left with an implanted post-hypnotic suggestion that may be harmful to themselves or others, explain that only suggestions that are consistent with their own values and beliefs will get through to their unconscious. Values and beliefs are extremely resistant to change and will certainly not yield to post-hypnotic suggestions that are inconsistent with them.

Build rapport and establish what the client wants to achieve

Be patient and listen carefully, asking all necessary questions to fully understand what the client wants to achieve. It will show your support and build rapport, which is crucial if the treatment is to work.

Suggestibility tests

The next thing is to do a series of suggestibility tests. Tell the client that being suggestible is very beneficial, because a suggestible person will be able to access their unconscious. The tests will provide an indication of the best induction method to use. Here is the first one:

The Postural Sway Test
The postural sway test will guide your client to become more responsive to you, rather than to their own thoughts. Say to the client

This is an exercise to test how well you can relax and concentrate. I want you to stand nice and straight. Keep your feet together. (Ensure their feet remain together throughout the exercise).That's right. Now close your eyes and turn your face up towards the ceiling, keeping your eyes closed. In a moment, you are going to feel as if you are falling backwards.

Test to check they are relaxed and not resisting by tipping them slightly backwards, but not enough for them to be aware you are doing so.

Don't worry. You're safe. I'm here to catch you if you do. Neither try to, nor resist falling. Just concentrate on my words and let yourself go whichever way your body wants to go. And I wonder if you notice that your body is actually swaying backwards and forwards, quite safely of course, as your unconscious mind will stop you going too far. Now you can stop imagining and open your eyes.

Point out to the client that this demonstrates that they are indeed suggestible.

Balloon test
Now go on to carry out the balloon test. Explain to your client that this is a quick test just to see how well they can focus on their own imaginings. Say to them:

Now I want you to stand upright, with your feet shoulder width apart. I want you to hold your arms straight out in front of you at shoulder height, palms downwards. And now I want you to close your eyes and turn your right hand over, palm upwards.

And now I want you to close your eyes and listen very carefully to what I say. I want you to imagine you have a heavy book on your right hand ... And it's so heavy that is trying to push your arm downwards... and you are trying to hold the book, but the weight of it is trying to push your arm down and down, and down. Now I want you to also imagine that a helium balloon is tied to your left hand ... And it's so light that it's trying to lift your left arm up ... and up ... and lifting ... lifting ... lifting ... upwards... and upwards.... The balloon is trying to pull your left arm upwards ... and the heavy book is trying to push your right arm downwards... It's feeling heavier and heavier... and the balloon in your left hand is feeling lighter ... and lighter. And now, keeping your hands in that position, I want you to open your eyes and look at them. Look where they are. If your arm moved from being parallel then you are suggestible and it means that your body will listen to suggestions from your unconscious, because that is what it has been doing to effect the changes in the position of your arms which you have now witnessed.

The finger vice test

Now move on to a third test - the finger vice test. Say to your client:

I want you to clasp your hands together like this, with the index fingers pointing upwards. Now separate the tips of your index fingers about an inch from each other and freeze this position, keeping the rest of your fingers firmly closed.

And now I want you to imagine there's a small vice around the tips of your index fingers. And now I'm going to turn the handle of the vice slowly ... and as I turn the vice handle the vice starts to close those fingers in towards each other ... Look at how your index fingers are closing."

Continue cranking the imaginary vice and verbalising as you go until the tips of your client's fingers are butted tightly together.

This test is the most powerful yet for convincing your client that they are suggestible, because, rather than just witnessing retrospectively what has happened, while they have had their eyes closed, here, they can witness it happening in front of their eyes, second by second.

Dealing with habitual contradictors

Occasionally, in the getting to know phase of the pre-induction interview you will become aware that your client is a habitual contradictor, a person who always disagrees. For example, if you say, "Good morning, and what a beautiful day" your client will respond with something like,

"Oh, I feel it's rather cold" and generally respond like that. In such a case, just reverse all the instructions for these tests. Ask them to do quite the opposite of what you want them to do. For example, in the balloon test, say to them:

Even though the balloon is pulling your left hand upwards and the book is weighing heavily down on your right hand you keep your hands steady and parallel. ... The balloon in your left hand continues to try to pull it upwards ... and the book on your right hand continues to press ... ever more heavily down ... heavily down ... and the balloon tied to your left hand continues to try to pull it upwards.

Similarly, in the vice test, say:

As I crank the handle, the vice applies pressure to the outside of the tips of your index fingers ... pulling them closer and closer together ... but your mind can resist it ... tighter and tighter the vice cranks them together ... harder and harder it is to keep them apart ... but you continue to do so ... Tighter and tighter ... closer and closer.

5

Investigating the Symptom History

Exploring and recording your client's personal history is an important part of the treatment protocol in hypnotherapy. It is the most immediate and most comprehensive resource that will be available to you to enable you to begin to understand their problem.

This task also gives you an opportunity to establish rapport with your client. Don't miss the opportunity. Use all your skills in this task. Building rapport means getting on the same wavelength, so that your client trusts you, feels comfortable with you and will open up. Careful and intelligent use of pacing, body language, attention, empathy and sympathy needs to be demonstrated.

The six general categories of analytical questions will serve to structure your enquiry, in order to achieve maximum understanding - who, what, when, where, how and why. As you talk with your client, you can home in on general answers to enquire, not just who generally, but who specifically, not just what in general, but what in particular. As you gather the information, you will begin to be given clues as to the best procedures to use to treat the condition.

You will be aware, from your professional understanding of psychological matters, that that which the client thinks is the problem may not be the real problem. There may, and probably will, be a problem on a higher level, unknown to your client. Most of our mental functioning is in the unconscious mind.

Ask your client to give you examples of the problem occurring and build up a picture. They may, indeed, be presenting with more than one problem and give you several examples of each, but from your more advanced understanding of such things you may deduce that they stem from a common, higher-level problem.

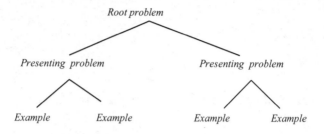

QUALITY OF INFORMATION

What a client tells you cannot be taken at face value. It may be true to the best of their understanding, but we all distort our experiences. This is because while about 2 million pieces of data present themselves for perception every second, our perceptual system can only handle a tiny proportion of them. In fact it is only 7±2 bits. There is, therefore, a large amount of selection going on and it is here where errors are made[23]. We make the selection by:

- deletion
- distortion
- generalisation

Deletion

We selectively pay attention to some bits of data and exclude other bits.

Distortion

We quickly distort the perception of particular experiences, to make them comparable with other experiences already stored in our memory, yet no two sets of circumstances are ever identical in reality. We also tend to often store a whole process of events as a single specific event, even though there was actually more to it than the specific event and the other parts may have had a significant effect upon us at an unconscious level.

The meta model

The meta model is a tool developed in the field of neurolinguistic programming (NLP) for spotting language patterns which indicate that the client is either intentionally, or unconsciously hiding information.

---

[23] Marshall (2012f) Ch.1.

This model is the negative of the Milton model, which you will encounter later in the treatment chapter of this book. The latter seeks to introduce deletions, distortions and generalisations into the information the hypnotherapist presents to the client, so that they can correct for them. The meta model, in contrast, seeks to correct a client's deletions, distortions and generalisations in the information they present the hypnotherapist.

Deletions
Here is taxonomy of the kinds of deletions people make.

Nominalisations
These are nouns derived from verbs, e.g..

The therapist can enquire:

- "There is no understanding."

  - "Who is it that doesn't understand?"
  - "Who is it that is not understood?"
  - "What is it that is not understood?"

- "There is no respect"

  - "Who is it that doesn't respect?"
  - "Who is it that is not respected?"

Unspecified verbs
E.g. "She rejected me."

"How, exactly, did she reject you?"

Simple deletion
E.g. "I am unhappy."

"Who is it that you are unhappy about?"

Verbs without subjects
"They don't care."

"Who, exactly, is it that doesn't care?"

Comparative deletions, e.g.

Hypnotherapists response

- She is more capable

"More capable of what?"

"More capable than who?"

- better
- best
- cleverer
- more
- most

Distortions

Mind reading
This refers to when a person assumes
they know what their interlocutor is thinking, e.g. "You think I'm being silly"

"How do you know I think you're being silly?"

Lost performatives
These are general value judgements without a subject, e.g. "It is not proper to..."

"Who says?"

Cause and effect.
This category of distortions refers to wrong attribution of cause and effect, e.g. "He makes me upset."

"How does he make you upset?"
"What is it, specifically, that he does to make you upset?"

Complex equivalence
This category refers to statements that contain invalid, implied synonymity. In other words, where a person wrongly assumes one condition is necessarily associated with another. An example could be a statement such as:
"He's always criticising me. He thinks I'm stupid."

"How does criticising you show that he thinks you're stupid? Do you think everyone you criticise is stupid, or do you criticise some people whose behaviour you just disapprove of?"

"Don't people criticise people for reasons other than that they think they are stupid?"

Presuppositions
This category refers to assumptions (right or wrong) a person may make that a second person who did something to them knew, or did not know, what the inevitable, or probable consequences would be. An example could be:

"She made me feel so embarrassed. It shows how much she cares about how I feel"

How do you know she was aware of how she made you feel?

Generalisations
Imperative forms
This category refers to terms such as: have to, must, must not, should, should not.

What would happen if you didn't?
What would happen if you did?

Modal operatives
These are terms implying possibility, or impossibility

What would be the case if you could?
What if you couldn't?

Universal quantifiers
This category refers to the use of terms such as: all, every, everyone, everywhere, no one, never, etc.

The therapist can question the universality implied in their statement. Are they really using the right word? Ask what would happen if this were not the case

Listen carefully to your client's responses. You may spot remedies to their problem in the form of helping them to recover lost experiential information, which has resulted in, or exacerbated, their problem. The recovery of this may make large changes, or small changes that become generative. By the latter I am referring to the fact that positive changes can start small and generate other changes until a large positive change is achieved.

How to begin

You could begin by simply asking your client why he or she has come to see you. Then draw the client out by asking: "And is there any other reason?", and so on.

Get them to be specific, for example, if they say, "I can't speak in public", ask:

What prevents you from doing so? Follow this with questions like, *How, exactly, does it prevent you? What are the consequences, or effects upon you?*

Ask them to give you an example of their problem, in order that you can get more detail of their experience of it. This is important, particularly where conditions like panic attacks are concerned. Ask, also, whether there are particular times when the symptoms come on.

Ask them when the problem started and what events there were in their life leading up to the time the problem started.

Ask why they actually think they have a problem. It may, or may not, be that this is a condition that is normal to most people.

Ask them to describe to you what happened when the problem first occurred and encourage them to be specific by probing questions. Ask them how they felt at the time, what has happened since and how they have felt each time it has happened. Enquire as to what were the general and specific conditions of life at the time the problem started, the length of time the problem has been present and whether there was, during that time, ever a period when the problem was not present. If so, what were the general and specific conditions then? Were they different in any way?

Ask them to describe, on a scale of 1 to 10, how it affects their state of well-being and, on the same scale, how much it debilitates them in normal daily functioning.

Enquire, also, if appropriate, whether the problem has ever been investigated medically?

Establish the goal of hypnotherapy

You have to establish the goal of therapy and agree this with your client, so ask him, or her, exactly what it is they want to achieve through these sessions - how they want to change, and why. This will often require some negotiation, as some clients will have unrealistic expectations. This is why this part of the process is so important. If your client has unrealistic expectations your hypnotherapy is never going to achieve them. Your client will be dissatisfied, the hypnotherapy will fail, and the client may lose faith in hypnotherapy and, thereby, close the door on a means of resolving problems and improving well-being in the future.

Medical or physical conditions

Ascertain whether your client has any medical condition for which they are currently being treated and whether they are, or have ever been treated for a psychological condition. Ask them what steps they have taken up to now to resolve their problem. Have they discussed it with anyone else? Have they had professional counselling, guidance or other treatment for it? If so by whom?

Motivation for seeking resolution through hypnotherapy

Ask them what made them decide to seek a resolution through hypnotherapy. Enquire whether they have been hypnotised before. If so, ask when and by whom and ask them to describe the method used, why the hypnotherapist said he had use that method and whether it helped.

Is the client the cause or effect?

Try to find out whether your client appears to be the cause or the effect of the symptom he, or she, is describing, i.e. does he, or she, appear to be in control of events? You could ask, quite boldly, but gently, *When might you have created this problem for yourself?*

Ask them, *Does, or could the problem have a purpose for you?* You may need to follow this up with an explanation of what you mean, but your client may respond immediately without further explanation.

You might extend your enquiry as follows:

Could there be something that your unconscious is trying to communicate to you, some need that is not being fulfilled, which, if it was being fulfilled, would result in the problem going away?

A natural follow-on from this, that will strengthen rapport and the client's own involvement in the process, would be:

Do you think that your unconscious mind will support our actions today, to bring about relief and a resolution of this problem and to allow you to experience the problem disappearing as a result of the treatment?

The roots of psychological problems are invariably to be found in the client's childhood. It is in the early stages of this that errors of storage are most easily made. Before the age of about five the child's judgemental abilities are not developed enough to critically appraise incoming data or judge the validity and veridity of what their parents say to them. Therefore, data goes straight into the unconscious, unmodified by judgement of the consequences and, therefore, has its effects in the same undiluted way. This is why inhibitions our parents instilled in us then still affect our behaviour in adulthood, even if we know that they are no longer justified.

Indeed, these kinds of storages are so powerful that it is the same kind of storage that we hypnotists try to achieve. We can't make a person's judgemental faculties become immature again, but we can keep them busy, so that they don't notice the data going in, or so relaxed that they don't care. It's not quite as good, but effective nevertheless.

Start to explore their childhood and its relationship with the current problem. Just say, for example:

Now let's talk about your childhood. Tell me about your family. Do you have brothers and sisters?

Consider whether their relationship with each of these relates to their current problem.

Look out for a possible strategy they have for having this problem, the function that it serves for them. For example, has it enabled them to gain attention or avoid it? Has it enabled them to avoid facing up to another, more real problem? Thomas Hardy's novel, *The Woodlanders,* provides an example of this kind of thing, where an old man has a debilitating obsession about a tree falling on his home. When the doctor orders the tree to be felled the old man dies of a heart attack. The obsession about the tree had been obscuring from him the intolerability of his life and, with the tree gone, he is forced to face it and he cannot cope with it.

An old woman attended a smoking cessation clinic I held. Her health was seriously threatened and she had apparently tried several different methods to quit. She was more or less frogmarched into my room by her sons, one on each side. After talking to her it became clear that hypnotherapy would not work, because the health scares that her chain-smoking was causing was serving to make her family worry about her and this gave her their attention. If she quit smoking and her health improved she feared she would not have that attention.

This is what I mean by possible strategies the client may have, however, conscious, or unconscious.

Biographical details

At some point, you need to take their basic biographical details. This may have already been done if you have a receptionist. He or she may have given the client a questionnaire to fill in, or may have asked the client for the details. You need to record their name, address, date of birth, phone number, by whom they were referred, or from where they got your details.

Sensitive questions

You could do with knowing whether they are married, in a stable relationship, or single. This is important, because it could have an influence on their problem and the resolution. However, asking people if they are married can be tricky; the motive for asking can be misinterpreted and you have to ask sensitively. Clients may also fail to see how it is relevant and regard it as none of the therapist's business.

Use of a questionnaire can avoid embarrassment in this respect, as people routinely see such questions as normal in questionnaires. Such a question could be worded in a multiple-choice form, such as married/single/cohabiting*delete as applicable.

This would not be likely to cause a client any concern, while asking a member of the opposite sex if they are married or single might. In general, it's not what you ask that can offend, or not offend, it's how you ask it.

You need to ask them who is their GP. You might also ask about hobbies. You can glean important therapy resource ideas from this information. If their hobby is photography, their dominant sensory system is likely to be visual. If they say music it's likely to be auditory and if they say cooking, it's likely to be gustatory. This information can be used to create the most effective kinds of images and metaphors to aid induction, create trance phenomena and couch powerful suggestions.

For the same reason, and also, perhaps, to prevent inappropriate techniques being selected, you need to ask your client if they are sensitive to light, whether they are phobic about anything and whether they happy about being touched.

6

Gathering Therapy Resources

Utilisation of environmental stimuli

Utilisation of things that happen around you in an induction situation are both important and powerful. If you don't involve things like a clock ticking, a window shutter screeching, or a client's blinking, then these things will serve to keep the client anchored to the conscious world and work against a successful induction. Conversely, if you do intelligently utilise them, they will actually aid your efforts to induce a deep and successful induction and therapy. Involve them wisely and they will reinforce your efforts as if you had an assistant present adding another layer to your induction. It is important, therefore, to keenly gather a mental stock of all the resources you will be able to use in the session and, indeed, all those external stimuli that you would be unwise to ignore. What kinds of resources can be utilised?

Material things in the environment

Things on the walls that could be used as focal point, such as:

- A clock
- A picture
- A fire burning in the grate, or a gas flame
- Clouds outside the window in a blue sky
- Warmth (A client is unlikely to be able to be induced successfully if he, or she, is cold).
- A comfortable chair, preferably, but not essentially, a recliner with a footstool facility.

Predictable things that happened during an induction

- A clock ticking
- The sound of rain dripping
- Relaxing music

A ticking clock is very hypnotic. People find the ticking of a clock comforting and this can help take a person quickly into a trance.

Rain falling outside is not an ideal sound, but if it is there you have to live and work with it. You can use it to carry your suggestions, such as:

As the raindrops gently dribble down, so you also drift deeper and deeper into a comfortable and soothing trance.

Unexpected sounds
There will inevitably be, from time to time, unexpected noises, such as a motor vehicle passing outside, an aircraft passing overhead, a church bell ringing, the heating system bursting noisily into life, a dog barking, bird songs or, worse still, a knock on the door. You have to include these noises in your induction, or they will work against you, bringing your client out of the trance. You need to be ready to respond to them in a useful way.

If, for example, a helicopter passes overhead, you might say:

And as you now hear that aircraft passing gently by, conveying away the last of your tension with it and leaving you completely relaxed.

Another example is:

And you may feel almost pleasantly surprised that even that motor vehicle noise cannot disturb the calm relaxation you now feel.

The heating system bursting into life can be responded to with words such as:

And as you hear that noise, just think of it as your mind dumping the worry and neurotic obsession that has been troubling you.

A dog barking is unfortunate, but you can suggest that it is warning off, forever, the neurotic obsession that has been troubling the client.

The sound of bells ringing can be utilised with words like:

And it's as if the ringing of those bells can be the signal that you are ready to go comfortably into the trance. Add the assuring words: *That's right*, or, if you have already ended the therapy you can suggest that:

The bell is telling you that you have let this problem go. It has come to an end and it is time to move on to a new period of freedom from your pain.

Personal things about your client
Personal things about your client are useful therapy resources. For example, their beliefs, words they seem to like using, their personal history and even their neurotic habits all can be linked into the suggestions you make to them. They will make them more likely to be accepted because these linkings will make the suggestions familiar and less alien.

Physiological stimuli

One of the most useful resources in an induction is the client's own breathing. The way a client is breathing is highly visible to the therapist and they can utilise it to pace their words with the client's breathing rate, saying their words on each outbreath and keeping them in pace with them.

Moreover, they can gradually slow their words and slow the client's breathing rate by so doing. Not only can you influence the rate of breathing, but you can gradually smooth out any irregularity of breathing pattern, because of the client's tendency to mirror their breathing to the pace of delivery of your words.

Words such: as *That's right*, and *Deeply relaxed* are the right length to match out-breaths. The words, *That's right* should be used frequently, to reinforce the client behaviour that the therapist wants to induce. If you also induce the client to focus on their own breathing you will speed up the induction into a trance, as it turns the client's focus away from the external world, towards something inward and rhythmic

Blinking

Everyone blinks periodically and blinking will increase as a client approaches the trance. Blinking also occurs when a person is becoming tired and you can use this to gradually make a client believe they are becoming tired, with suggestions like:

And you are aware that your eyes are blinking ... your eyelids becoming heavy and tired ... ever more tired ... heavy and tired ... so that they are wanting to close.... That's right, Let them close.

A person's breathing pattern changes as they approach sleep and you can usefully pace a client into a breathing pattern that is present in a state approaching sleep - a hypnagogic state.

Swallowing is an indicator that the client is moving into a trance state. This is a resource that you can use as a gauge of how deep the client is in the induction process.

Utilise the feelings in the client's limbs

The client's own awareness of their own hypnotic behaviour is a very powerful convincer of their own suggestibility, so utilise procedures like the arm catalepsy procedure and make the client aware of what their arm is doing.

As you convince the client that they are becoming ever more relaxed, perhaps in the process of progressive muscle relaxation, you can instruct them to feel their muscles becoming relaxed and heavy. Making a client's arm move upwards by hypnosis is a powerful convincer of a client's ability to be hypnotised. You can enhance the process by asking the client to be alert to muscle twitches and elbow creaks. For example:

And as your arm gradually starts to lift itself up all by itself ... you may become aware of the start of a gentle movement ... perhaps a muscle twitching ... or an elbow creaking...

Space and comfort as a resource

Another resource you need to utilise is the space available. You need to position yourself in relation to your client so that a balance is struck between infringement of personal space and sufficient proximity to observe the client's breathing pattern and other physiological clues to their inner state.

You can utilise the softness of the chair in which the client is sitting. For example, you can say:

And as you sink ever more deeply into the comfort of that chair.

The fact that the client will be conscious of their surroundings may cause them to doubt that they are actually under hypnosis and may, indeed, serve to anchor them to the non-trance state. They have to be awake for the induction to work.. If they were asleep it would not and if they are awake they will be aware of their surroundings. If you inform them of this in advance you will forestall this drawback.

7

Induction Techniques

There are various ways of inducing trance that range from the most permissive to the most authoritarian. The best induction method to use, most of the time is the one you like best, but you must be prepared to switch, as no technique will work for everyone. Highly analytical clients, for example, will not respond so well to deep relaxation but may be induced more successfully by confusion techniques.

You can, in fact, move straight from the suggestibility tests into induction if you feel it is appropriate. It is usual, however, for a hypnotherapist to spend some time building rapport first, as clients will only let go when trust between them and the hypnotherapist has been established.

Postural sway induction
The postural sway induction is form of induction that can be performed immediately following the postural sway suggestibility test, if you wish. When you feel the client falling back into your hands, carry the movement smoothly through, conveying your client gently into a chair with the reassuring words:

That's right. Let go. All the way now. Just let yourself go deeper ... and deeper asleep ... feeling those wonderful relaxation feelings washing over you ... as you sleep deeply ... and comfortably.

Facilitating a naturally occurring trance
The general principle here is that you have to give their conscious mind something absorbing to do, imagining a tranquil scene, or an enjoyable event they have had, or would like to have.

As they focus their mind inwards, look carefully at trance analogies and reinforce them with words like, *That's right, Deeper, All the way through, relaxing you.*

Pacing current experience

Pacing current experience involves directing the client's attention to a small number of external stimuli, which he or she can verify and add a suggestion about internal awareness, for example:

And as you sit comfortably in that chair... listening to my voice and feeling your feet firmly on the floor...so you are feeling more and more relaxed.

Now repeat the process, utilising two or three different external stimuli, for example: The sound of the breeze outside the window, my voice and the comfort of that chair", and add some more words about internal comfort and relaxation and suggestions that your client is sliding deeper and deeper into the trance.

Continue with the process, decreasing the number of external stimuli suggestions and increasing the number of suggestions about internal feelings. Change your voice gradually from normal everyday speaking manner to a monotonic, hypnotic voice, as you progress towards a stage where all your suggestions are about internal feelings.

Here, for example, the only reference to external stimuli is the ticking of the clock.

And as you hear the gentle tick of the clock, so you feel your whole body beginning to relax and you are entering the trance.

Repeat the process again and maybe even again, depending on how deeply you perceive your client is entranced, progressively lowering your voice and increasing its monotonic tone until all the suggestions are about internal state rather than external stimuli.

Revivification

The revivification induction method involves getting your client to relive a past experience - one in which they were very absorbed at the time.

1.   Casually bring up an event and then say, for example:
        What's it like to be really absorbed in that event?

2.   Use the meta model to ask further details, i.e. who, what, when, where, how and why.

3.   Follow on from these answers to ask what happened next. Use connectives, such as: so, with, while, since, after, then.

4.   Gradually change the terms of the dialogue from past to present and their focus of attention from external to internal events, for example:
        So you are sitting on the riverbank, feeling calm. ... And do

you feel relaxed?

5.   Identify and remember key trance words and/or phrases the client uses and repeat them, using the client's intonation, as much as you can.

The conscious/unconscious dissociation method of inducing a trance

This method of inducing a trance involves alternately talking to the client about the conscious and unconscious minds, using different voice qualities for each, for example, speaking in a normal voice, say:

The conscious mind works in a logical, sequential and linear way...

Then, in your monotonic, hypnotic voice, add:

...while the unconscious works spatially and intuitively.

Follow this in your normal voice again, saying:

Your conscious mind is processing by words and numbers.

Then add, in your hypnotic voice:

...while your unconscious mind is using images and feelings

Returning to your normal voice again, say:

While your conscious mind analyses,

Follow, in your hypnotic voice, with:

... your unconscious mind understands, feels and uses metaphor, imagery and symbol.

You can further distinguish between these two voices by changing the position from which you speak, for example, by the side of your client for the everyday voice and from behind the client for the hypnotic voice, or any other variation of this you wish to try.

Eye fixation

Fixation on a single thought induces a trance. James braid discovered this in 1843. He also discovered that fixation upon the eyes causes fatigue of the eyelid, leading to eyelid exhaustion. When this occurs, clients are unable to open their eyes. These effects are the basis of the eye fixation induction technique.

1.   Ask your client to sit comfortably in a chair with their feet flat on the floor and their hands by their sides.

2.   Ask them to look at a spot on the wall, or some other object above the level of their eyes, raising only their eyes to do so - not their head. This will stimulate alpha waves in the brain.

3. Direct your client to: *Concentrate exclusively on that object
    to the complete exclusion of everything else, as your eyes
    begin to become ever more tired.*

Continue as follows.

4. *And as you continue focusing on that spot ... so your eyes are
    becoming ever more tired ... heavy and tired ... and so they
    are wanting to close. And as you continue to focus on that
    spot ... your eyes are beginning to close ... so let them
    comfortably close.*

5. *Do the eyelid fixation, suggestibility test by placing your
    finger on the client's forehead and moving it up to the top of
    the head. Watch to see if your client's eyeballs move
    upwards, inside their eyelids, thus confirming their
    suggestible state.*

6. *Proceed from there to deepen the trance, using whatever
    deepeners you feel are appropriate.*

Re-induction anchors
The re-induction anchor is post-hypnotic cue implanted in a previous
session, for the purpose of rapidly inducing trance at a subsequent
time. It goes without saying, then, that this cannot be used to induce a
trance the first time you meet your client.
   Various things can be used as reinduction anchors, for example:
shoulder squeezes, finger clicks, or simple words.

How to implant a re-induction anchor.

1. While the client is entranced, compliment them on their
    ability to enter the trance rapidly and deeply. Say, for
    example, "You are an excellent hypnotic subject and can
    easily enter a trance and to make things easier still, whenever
    I touch you on the shoulder like this (touch their shoulder)
    you will immediately re-enter the trance and go comfortably
    as deep, or even comfortably deeper.

2. Repeat three or four times.

3. Awaken the client, allow them to reorientate themselves and
    then test the anchor works by touching them on the shoulder
    in the manner you suggested. It's unlikely to happen

instantly. You'll notice some trance analogue phenomena, such as defocusing, or glazing over of the eyes.

4.   Reinforce this with words such as, "That's right. Go all the way down ... deeply and comfortably back into the trance ... all the way down ... deeper and deeper."

Rapid induction techniques
Rapid inductions require the right circumstances to be set up. A *yes set* should be carried out first, which can be induced by means of a series of successful tests of suggestibility.

Rapid inductions depend essentially on:

- surprise, confusion and overload
- trance analogue reinforcement

Confusion is a doorway into the unconscious, where the ego goes to escape while it resolves confusion. When this happens, reinforce by commanding your client to:

Go into a trance! Sleep! Then watch for every trance analogue and reinforce each with words like: *That's right ... Just let yourself go deeper ... comfortably deeper, Let those wonderful waves of relaxation surround you, as you go deeper.*

The movement from the state of confusion to one of increasing relaxation will induce a deepening trance.

The handshake rapid induction
This is the famous Ericksonian handshake induction. It uses confusion from an interrupted, normal handshake.

1.   Go to shake hands with your client in the normal way. You must, yourself, at this stage, act as if you are going to shake hands normally, so that it happens as a natural gesture and not a trick.

2.   Stop the movement just before your hands touch and, instead, gently take hold of the client's wrist with your left hand and, pointing to the palm with your right index finger, look surprised and say: *Look.*

3.   Look curiously and intently at their hand until they also begin to look at it.

4.   Say: *Can you see those lines and shadows over there, in that hand, as your mind relaxes ... and now ... closing your eyes only as quickly as you can allow that comfort to spread...*

5.   Add some deepening suggestions.

Induction by specific eye fixation with relaxation
Say to your client:
Do you see that point up there on the ceiling?
Point to the spot
   I want you to focus your eyes upon it.... And as you continue to look at it steadily for a while... I would like you just to listen to what I say... paying full attention to that point on the ceiling... my words and whatever else I may ask you to attend to.... Even if your eyes should wander from that point... that will be all right... just bring your eyes back to it.... And in a few moments you may notice changes as you continue to look at that point...It may move or change colour. It may get bigger or smaller... or get blurry... vanish... come back or vanish altogether....Or it may do something different. Whatever it does or does not do will be fine. Just watch and let it happen.
   And while you watch that point ... I wonder if you can begin to notice the relaxation that is beginning to take place in your body... especially in your feet. Your feet are beginning to relax... the muscles of your right foot are relaxing... and those of your left foot... relaxing too.... And now the relaxation is spreading up... to your calf muscles... the left one... and the right one... and on up to your thighs... You are becoming increasingly relaxed as you keep watching that point. ...The fingers of your right hand are becoming relaxed... and now your left hand.... The relaxation is going up into the muscles of your left forearm... and those of your right forearm... your stomach muscles are relaxing too... and now your upper arms... and your chest muscles.... On up through your neck muscles... you can notice, too how your back muscles and your shoulder muscles are becoming relaxed.... Your whole body is becoming relaxed... more and more relaxed... including the muscles of your face... of your scalp.... And now you notice, or perhaps you have already noticed, that there is a heaviness in your feet.... Your feet and your legs are becoming heavy... your hands and your arms are heavy... your whole body is heavy... pleasantly heavy...And you can notice particularly how h-e-a-v-y your eyelids have become... In fact, the whole of your body has become drowsy and sleepy... very drowsy,... your eyelids heavy.... Your eyes are tired from staring at that point... Your eyes want to blink.
   Once they start blinking, continue with:
Your eyes are blinking ... and blinking again ... more ... and ... more.

Your utterance of the word *more* should be synchronised with the client's actual, physical blinks.

Each time you blink it gets harder for your eyes to open.... Your eyes are clo-sing... clo-sing.... Soon they will close completely.... Your eyelids are getting heavier and heavier.... Your eyes are closing, clo-sing... more and more.... They are so heavy... you can hardly keep them open.... Your eyes are nearly closed... .In a few moments they will close completely ... all on their own... and... remain closed.

When your client's eyes are closed, reinforce the suggestion. Say: *That's right. ... Keep them closed.*

In the unlikely event that your client's eyes are still open at this point you will need to instruct them firmly to close them. Say, for example: *That's right. Just close your eyes now! Close them! Keep them closed.*

The arm catalepsy induction technique
This is a mildly authoritarian induction technique. Say to your client:

I want you to sit comfortably, with your feet flat on the floor and your hands on your lap, palms upwards. And I want you to focus on your left hand (or right hand, whichever you choose).

Take hold of your client's wrist gently with your thumb and forefinger, where the wrist meets the hand. Gently lift and lower the hand until you perceive a cataleptic state has occurred in the wrist. This movement is very gentle. To describe it as a gentle shake would probably be to overstate it, but, inversely, to describe it simply as an up-and-down movement would be to understate it. It is somewhere between these two actions.

When you sense a cataleptic state has been achieved (when the arm seems to be prepared to remain raised on its own) release your client's wrist and proceed to guide their hand up by gentle, diagonal strokes underneath, with your thumb and forefinger alternately.

When your client's hand has reached the level of their face, say:

I want you to continue to see that hand, right there in your mind's eye, even after your close your eyes.... Let them close... and as soon as you're ready... both on the conscious and unconscious level... to allow the whole of your body to relax,... for the whole of your body to continue to relax much more deeply... than you have experienced in a long while... that hand... with slow, unconscious, gentle movements... can gradually begin to drift down to your lap...

The eye roll induction
To induce by the eye roll method, say to your client:

And when you are ready to enter the trance... I would like you to... comfortably... close your eyes... and with your eyelids comfortably closed... I would like you to allow your eyes to roll back... as if you were focusing on a spot at the back of your mind... and in a few moments I want you to try and open those eyes while you continue to focus fully on that spot... and the harder you try to open those eyes the tighter closed they will become.... In fact, while you focus on that spot it will become impossible for those eyes to open ... and when you are sure there is no way that they could open I would like you to test them.

Authoritarian induction

An authoritarian induction technique works best with compliant subjects, or those who are used to obeying orders, such as military personnel. It is particularly appropriate where rapid induction is needed, for example, where a person is in severe pain.

Say to your client:

As you look at that spot you will relax quickly and deeply (10 second pause). *Your legs will grow heavy ... very heavy (10 second pause). Your arms will grow heavy ... very heavy* (10 second pause). *Your entire body will grow heavy ... very heavy* (10 second pause). *And now your legs are heavy, your arms are heavy and your entire body is heavy...* (10 second pause). *Your eyes are now growing heavy .... They are becoming tired ... very tired. You will want to close your eyes.... As you close your eyes, you will go deeply asleep.*

It's important to carefully watch the condition and movement of your client's eyes as you perform this induction procedure.

Continue with:

Your eyes are growing heavier all the time. They are closing... closing... closing.... They are so very heavy and tired.... As your vision distorts... so you want to close your eyes....It's so difficult to keep them open.... Closing... closing... closing.

About 70% of clients will close their eyes at this time. If this doesn't happen, repeat the process for a few minutes. If they still have not closed them command them to do so by saying:

Close your eyes please! If a client is deeply in a hypnotic trance by now, with their eyes open, which is not to be expected, but sometimes happens, you should just gently close their eyelids with your fingers.

Continue as follows.

Deep, deep asleep... deep, deep, asleep.... Repeat these words four or five times, at two or three second intervals. This will narrow their focus down to a single idea - that of being deep, deep asleep.

The emergency eye gaze induction

The emergency eye gaze induction is an alternative to the latter technique. It's the same except for the fact that here you direct the client to focus on your left, or right eye. Make sure you do not return the focus, though, or it will be you that goes into a trance, rather than the client. You should be looking straight ahead, not into the eyes of the client.

Permissive induction

At the opposite end of the scale is the permissive induction. This is more appropriate where clients are highly uncompliant. Proceed as follows.

And in your own time... I would like you to make yourself comfortable ... placing your feet flat on the floor... and allowing your palms to rest comfortably on your lap.... And when you are ready to begin some important inner work... and for the whole of your body to relax ... just gently allowing your eyes to close... and with your eyes comfortably closed ... becoming so much more aware of your breathing... so that with every in-breath you can breathe in a deep feeling of comfort and ease ... and all the while ... with each out-breath breathing out any unnecessary tension as we go on.

Advanced mind-body dissociation technique

This technique induces a client into a trance by creating confusion to keep the conscious mind busy, while the hypnotist addresses their unconscious. Proceed as follows.

And in a few moments time... you will hear me count down from ten to one... and with each descending number... between ten and one... the whole of your body will drift... one tenth deeper into the wonderful trance state... ten percent deeper asleep... deep sleep... sleeping... deeply... and independently from your mind... but of course not the usual sleep of bedtime... but a sleep in which your body can rest quite separately and aside from your mind... while at the same time you will also hear me... count up from one to ten... and with each ascending number... between one and ten... the whole of your mind will become... one tenth more alert... receptive... and focused ... on ideas and thoughts rushing through your mind"

Repeat the whole induction, from the beginning, a second time and then continue as follows.

So ready? ... Ten... your body... going deeper.... One... Your mind more alert.... Nine... Two... Eight... Three. Your mind more alert... Seven, Your body going... deeper asleep... Four... Six... Five... Five... Six... Four.... Your body deeper and deeper asleep... Seven. Your mind more alert... more focused.... Three... Eight... Two... Nine... And one.... The whole of your body... deep... deep... asleep.... And ten. Your mind so alert... receptive and focused. (30-second pause).

8

Deepening Techniques

Deeping by counting

Deeping by counting is a common method of deepening a trance. Say, for example:

In a moment I'm going to count ... from one to ten ... and with each number I count between one and ten ... you will become twice as deeply relaxed as you are now.... With each new number ... your level of feeling of comfort and peace will double ... so that by the count of ten you will be deeply and comfortably relaxed.

Begin counting, and with every three or four counts add a deepener suggestion, for example: *One ... Two ... Three ... and going deeper and deeper.... Four ... Five ...Six ... more comfortable and relaxed. Seven ... Eight ... Nine ... letting go.* Add confusion, such as skipping a number, overlapping a count, or reversing the numbers. Confusion will cause their focus to increasingly escape towards the peace and tranquillity of the unconscious.

On the count of ten, Say something like,

"You are now all the way down into a state of deep relaxation."

Direct suggestion

Instead of counting to the client, you can suggest that the client deepen their own trance by describing what it feels like to go into a trance, perhaps by reliving a pleasant memory.

Deepening by progressive relaxation

A particularly effective way of deepening a trance is by guided, progressive relaxation. Here is such a script that I was taught in my initial training:

And with your eyes comfortably closed... taking a moment... just to become aware of your breathing... so that with each out-breath. You can begin to breathe out any unnecessary nervous tension... and with each in-breath ... you can breathe in a deepening feeling of comfort and ease.... So as you allow that process to continue ... all by itself... I wonder if you can imagine a very peaceful or tranquil scene... or maybe a pleasant memory from the past... or somewhere relaxing you would like to visit... that reminds you of the wonderful feeling of being deeply relaxed ... And as you imagine that peaceful, tranquil scene... ever more clearly... just becoming aware of how much more relaxed your eyelids have naturally become... comfortably closed... and as you continue to experience that peaceful and tranquil scene... allowing those comforting feelings of relaxation to spread out from your eyelids... and into all of the muscles around your eyes... just allowing every muscle around your eyes to relax... deeply... and then beginning to experience that wonderful wave of, perhaps, warm relaxation ... gradually spreading out and through the muscles of your face... every muscle beginning to relax... and letting go... experiencing that wonderful wave of relaxation, spreading out into the muscles of your cheeks... and around your nose... every muscle just relaxing and letting go... as you enjoy that wonderful wave of relaxation, spreading up across your forehead... releasing any unwanted tension... and down through your mouth ... and your jaw... every muscle in your face just relaxing and letting go... as you enjoy that wonderful wave of relaxation ... spreading back across your scalp... and all the way back through your mind... every muscle just relaxing... and throughout every part of your mind... and now just allowing that warm feeling of deep relaxation to begin to spread... down from your face and scalp... and all the way down through your neck... every muscle just relaxing and letting go... and as you continue to imagine that very peaceful, tranquil scene... that wonderful wave of relaxation can begin to spread down into your shoulders... every muscle just relaxing and letting go... as that wave of relaxation begins to spread down through your upper arms and down through your chest... with each out-breath... just breathing out any unnecessary nervous tension... breathing freely and easily... as that wonderful wave of warm relaxation spreads down through your elbows... and into your forearms... every muscle just relaxing and letting go... and now... that wonderful wave of relaxation is spreading down through your wrists... and into your hands... every muscle just relaxing and letting go... as that wonderful wave of relaxation spreads all the way down through your fingers, to your fingertips.... You may even begin to experience your arms feeling so heavy... pushing down into your lap... your arms are feeling so heavy and tired... as you become aware of that deepening feeling of safety and relaxation spreading down into your stomach... every muscle just relaxing... and letting go... all the while the muscles from the top of your shoulders ... all the way down through your lower back are relaxing and letting go... and you can sink ever more deeply into the comfort of my chair... and as you continue to fully experience... that peaceful tranquil place... just allowing that wave of relaxation to spread down through your abdomen... and enjoying every muscle relaxing and letting go... so that the... whole top half of your body can begin to feel so comfortably... heavy... tired... and now just observing that wonderful wave of deep relaxation spreading... down through your waist... and into your thigh muscles... so that once again those muscles can begin to feel so comfortably heavy... every muscle relaxing and letting go.... And as you continue to breathe... ever more deeply and easily... so that wave of relaxation is spreading down through your knees... and into your calf muscles... that warm wave of relaxation helping every muscle to relax and let go... so that your legs can also feel so comfortably heavy too ... and then just allowing that wave of relaxation to spread... all the way down through your ankles... and into your feet... every muscle just relaxing and letting go... every muscle from the ends of your fingertips... to the tips of your toes... just relaxing and letting go... all the while enjoying... the feelings of safety and comfort that come from your own inner tranquil place.

Fractionalisation

Fractionalisation involves inducing a series of mini trances and bringing the client out of each one before inducing the next one. Each time a client goes into a trance it will be a bit deeper than the last time, because their mind is learning to enter the trance. Therefore, by inducing a series of mini trances the client goes deeper than if you just induce a single one. This is how to do it:

1. Induce a trance by whatever method you choose.

2. Bring the client out of the trance. Say, *In a moment I'm going to count backwards from three to one, but you are only to waken as quickly as you can go back into the trance when I touch you on the shoulder like this. So when I touch you on the shoulder like this you will immediately close your eyes and go as deeply into the trance as this, or even deeper.* (Touching the client on the shoulder, thus, becomes a re-induction anchor).

3. Repeat this two or three times, to make it clear to the client.

4. Count slowly backwards from three to one and wait for your client to open their eyes and begin to reorientate themselves, but before they have fully done so touch their shoulder and reinforce with the suggestion: *Going all the way down, deep inside the relaxing trance.*

5.   Repeat these steps until the client is as deeply entranced, as you wish them to be.

On each subsequent awakening, the client will be increasingly slow to begin to reorientate themselves and will sink increasingly deeper on each invocation of the reinduction anchor.

Here is an alternative script you can use, which I was taught in my own initial training.

And I will wake you in a few moments time... and when you are awake... we will talk for a little while... you will then hear me click my fingers like this... (Click your fingers)... *and when you hear me click my fingers like this...* (click your fingers again)... *your eyes will close... and you will go back into this deep state of relaxation... this deep ... inner state... and you will be just as deeply relaxed... just as deeply comfortable... as you are now... and you will only respond to this signal here... in this room... sitting in that chair... and you will never respond to this signal from anyone else... only to me... and only in this room... sitting in that chair... and when you are comfortable about entering the trance...*

What you can use as re-induction anchors

You can use any sign, in any modality, as a deepening anchor, although words and physical sensations are most commonly used. Just suggest to the entranced client that when they hear a particular word or phrase, or feel a particular physical sensation, for example, a touch on the shoulder, that they will go deeper into the trance

Some of the most common deepening anchors are:

- The *Nowww* word.
- A Squeeze of the shoulder
  (See previous page for an example)
- Hand drop
    Say for example. *In a moment, I'm going to lift your hand and let it fall onto your lap ... and every time you feel it fall onto your lap. You will go deeper into the trance.*
- Head rotation
    Say, for example: *In a moment I'm going to gently move your head like this.... and when I move your head gently like this ... you will go deeper and deeper relaxed.*
- Forehead touch.
    Say, for example, *In a moment I'm going to touch your forehead like this (gently touch your client's forehead, with enough pressure to lift it slightly) ... and when I*

touch your forehead like this (touch their forehead again)
... you will become even more deeply relaxed.

The hand levitation deepener

The hand levitation deepener is designed to be used in conjunction
with the arm catalepsy induction. (See p.63).

Ask your client to look at one of their hands and say:

As you continue to look at that hand... it's perfectly natural... that
your vision will distort... but what I really want you to pay attention
to... is the feelings... the physical sensations of the hand... any part of
the hand.... You may notice a slight tremor in one of the fingers... or
the thumb.... There may be a slight movement of the whole hand... as
an elbow contracts.... You may experience a wooden like sensation in
the back of the hand.... And it really doesn't matter what feelings
develop in that hand... the important thing for you to do... is to sense
fully... whatever sensations develop... and in a few moments time... I
will ask your inner mind... to allow your hand to feel... very, very
light... and... your unconscious mind to lift that hand off your lap....
And you can find that hand will feel lighter and lighter all the time...
and the lifting... can occur slowly... hesitantly... the movement will be
slow... and uncertain.... And all I want you to notice is... how ... with
each breath you are taking in... your hand is lifting... lifting just a
little bit... just floating into the air ... as if attached to a large
balloon... lifting higher and higher... becoming lighter and lighter all
the time... lifting... lifting... lifting.... You may find it more comfortable
to even allow your eyes to close... as you observe that experience
beginning to develop all by itself.

When you client's hand has reached almost shoulder level continue
with the deepener as follows:

And when your inner mind is ready to allow you to drift... perhaps a
hundred times more deeply into the trance... that hand can begin to
feel so heavy... so very heavy... as if you have let go of that balloon...
and with every millimetre that hand drifts down towards your lap... so
you are becoming ever more deeply relaxed... that you just drift ever
more deeply into your own inner experience... and... your hand can
now slowly return to your lap... and with every millimetre of the way
down... you are going deeper and deeper relaxed... all the way deep
down and relaxed ... and when your hand reaches your lap... it will
rest there (insert your client's name here)... *comfortably rest there ...*
and that hand will only reach your lap as soon as your mind gently
begins to drift... to wonder... or to dream

The countdown deepener

Once your client has closed their eyes say:

And you may have already noticed how your breathing has changed... And as we go on ... with each in-breath... you can breathe in a deeper feeling of comfort and ease... and with each out-breath... you can breathe out any unnecessary nervous tension.... And as you do this, you can go deeper into the wonderful state of hypnotic relaxation. And as we go on... you can go ... d-e-e-p-e-r (say the word as the client breathes out)... d-e-e-p-e-r (say the word as the client breathes out)... *and still   ...*   d-e-e-p-e-r (say the word as the client breathes out). *In a few moments time... you will hear me countdown from ten to one ... and with each descending number... between ten and one... you are going to become one tenth more relaxed... ten percent more relaxed... with each descending number.... Each descending number... will help you to go one tenth deeper... into that wonderful... hypnotic, inner state of relaxation... that naturally... will become deeper and deeper... as you go on... and if... while I'm counting... you will experience a slight... though pleasant... physical sensation... as if you were floating... floating down... that will be fine.... It only means that you are drifting... into an ever-deepening state... of physical as well as mental relaxation.... And as you continue to explore your own creative, inner world... I would like you to know that you are always in control... and that you will go deeper... and deeper... as we go on....   So ready?... Ten, Nine ... and deeper and deeper... really enjoying just drifting... drifting down... Eight... Seven... Six... That's right, (insert your client's name here).... Ever more deeply relaxed... Five... Four.... And I wonder how soon it will be before your mind occasionally drifts or wanders.... Three... and deeper and deeper still.... Two... One... and all a way deep down... relaxing in your own inner experience...*

The stairs deepening technique

Here is another gentle deepener, which gives the client a bit of help to get their imagination going.

I would like you to imagine... that you are standing on a beautiful balcony... and there's a long staircase ... leading down from the balcony... and there is ... as yet ... no need for you to see ... where the stairs are leading to.... And they are strong stairs... with wide steps... and a handrail too, ... well lit... so that you can see clearly.... And in a few seconds time... I'm going to count down from ten to one ... but this time... with each descending number... not only do you go deeper relaxed ... but you can take a single step down... from the balcony....

And you will feel a curious sense of excitement with each step down the way... and when you reach step one... I will ask you to pause for a while... and you can wonder... where you are going next.... I will then ask you to step off... and when you do... you will find yourself in your favourite place of relaxation.... So ready? ... Take that first step down... Ten... Nine... and another step down... Eight... Seven and perhaps even feeling those feet just floating above a step... Six... and it's so nice to enjoy walking down... Five... Four... Three... and... another step... another step down... Two... One... and resting... wondering... where you will go next... (ten second pause) and you can... step off... and into your very own favourite place of relaxation... and enjoy... that wonderful place where you can take a long refreshing rest...

The elevator deepening technique

Here is another deepener script of this kind.

Imagine that you are seated in a comfortable chair in an elevator.... You're on the tenth floor... and you're seated so that you can see the hand on the dial ... that points to the numbers of the floors ... as you pass them.... The elevator moves very slowly... so the hand moves slowly from ten down towards nine.... You are nearing the ninth floor and you become quite drowsy... As the elevator moves downwards... you go deeper and deeper into your own inner world.... When you reach the ninth floor... you'll become more pleasantly and comfortably relaxed ... than you have been in a long while.... Now you reach and pass the ninth floor ... and the dial is slowly moving towards eight.... You become more and more relaxed... every sound that you hear... every easy breath that you take makes you go deeper ... deeper into drowsy relaxation.... The dial passes eight ... going down ... deeper and deeper... every muscle and every nerve relaxes as you see the hand passing seven.... So sleepy.... So perfectly comfortable... (short pause).... Now, you reach the sixth floor.... All of your cares and tensions are fading away as you go down ... down further into drowsy relaxation.... The hand is now at five... halfway down.... Let go more and more.... Let your mind relax also.... Just think of the hand on the dial as it moves on down to four... (short pause).... The hand is passing four, and as it passes... you let go again. Any unnecessary tension has almost completely disappeared... (short pause).... Three.... Almost there.... So relaxed... S-o-h sleepy.... The hand reaches two.... Now you're almost down to the first floor... where you can drift off... into a pleasant dream... or any other comforting experience you wish.... When the hand reaches one... the elevator doors will open and you can step out into your own, inner, favourite place of tranquillity.... And as you step out of that lift you can leave any last bit of tension

*behind.... So now that hand reaches one and those doors slide open...
and you can... step out... and into your very own, favourite place of
tranquillity... and enjoy... this wonderful place where you can take a
long, refreshing, inner rest.*

Out of body experience method

This dissociation method is powerful and useful, particularly where a
client is very resistant. It works by separating the functioning of the
conscious and unconscious parts of the mind. Here is a typical
example of a dissociation script, which I was taught when I first
trained and which I have used very successfully since. Both the
induction and the deepener are included here, as they are really
inseparable – you would not use the induction part without the deeper,
nor vice versa.

The induction part

*And only as soon as you're ready to begin some important inner work
I would like you to allow your eyes to close.... And with those eyes
comfortably closed... I would like you to take a few moments, just to
become fully aware of yourself ... your physical position ... resting
comfortably in my chair... and your position within the room...
perhaps noticing the support of my chair behind your back... and your
feet resting comfortably upon the floor... and the temperature of the
air around the skin of your face... as your breathing deepens.... And I
would like to give you an opportunity to explore your own inner
creative imagination.... I would like you to imagine that ... with each
in-breath ...you are feeling lighter and lighter... and in your own time
... that you are beginning to float... floating out of your physical
body... floating up into the air...*

The deepener part

*And looking down at your physical body ... resting so comfortably in
my chair... notice how you seem from above.... Then perhaps
floating... over to a corner of the room... so that you can view yourself
from a different perspective... observing your physical body relaxing,
ever more deeply.... And then allowing yourself to float down... just
above my carpet... and noticing how your physical body appears
different as you look up at yourself... and then just allowing yourself
to continue floating upwards... drifting slowly around my room... just
observing your physical body... becoming so much more relaxed... in
my chair ... and then floating down to rest in a different chair as we
go on.*

Ask your client to confirm, by a nod of the head, whether they have experienced this and now feel they are in a different chair, looking at themselves in another chair. When you have received such verification, proceed with your chosen therapy method.

After the therapy, it is vitally important to reintegrate your client. The way to do this will be described on page 135.

9

Discovering The Problem

Even if the client thinks they know the cause of their problem the unconscious is likely to be a more reliable source. To access this proceed as follows.

Induce a deep trance. Ask your client to verbalise their responses. If they don't do so, then use the ideomotor responding protocol. For this you need to ask your client to designate *Yes, No* and *Don't know* fingers.

The seven psychodynamics of neurotic symptoms.
Charles Tebbit identified seven psychodynamics of a symptom:

- Imprinting
- Unresolved current issue
- Secondary gain
- Identification
- Inner conflict.
- Past experience
- Self-punishment, or punishment of someone else

Imprinting
An imprint, in this context, is a stubborn belief instilled by an authority figure.

Unresolved current issue
Once uncovered by hypnosis an unresolved current issue can be dealt with consciously, albeit, perhaps, with enhanced willpower, as a result of the application of ego strengthening techniques and suggestion.

Secondary gain
There may be a secondary gain that your client is receiving as a result of their symptoms. Remember the client I mentioned earlier, the old

lady who had come to me to help her quit smoking. She was accompanied by her two sons, both of whom were very worried about the way her smoking was causing her health to deteriorate. She insisted she was incapable of giving up, despite the effect on her health.

It became clear to me that her inability to quit, despite the effect on her health, gained her the sympathy of her sons' attention that she craved in her otherwise lonely existence. A family therapy session was the best way of resolving this one.

If you think this kind of thing underlies your client's symptoms, find out, by verbalisation, or ideomotor responses, the nature of the secondary gain from the symptom/s.

You can also age regress to the first time the secondary gain was achieved, perhaps using the *affect bridge technique*, to go back to the origin.   Age regression and the affect bridge technique will be explained shortly.

Identification

A client's symptoms may be due to them unconsciously copying the behaviour of someone else, whom they admire .

Verbalisation under hypnosis might reveal this. If it is found to be the case, relay it back to the client, under hypnosis and they may see how inappropriate it is. Once such an unconscious cause is discovered it can be dealt with consciously, perhaps with the assistance of suggestion and ego strengthening.

Inner conflict

Many neurotic illnesses, for example obsessions and irrational fears, are created by the unconscious mind to deflect the sufferer's attention from a threatening and perceivably insoluble problem. Resolve one and you have to face a worse one. Such a neurosis needs to be resolved, because if the masked problem is a real threat it won't go away and threatens the individual's well-being in a real, rather than imaginary way

I gave the example in chapter 4 that occurred in Thomas Hardy's novel, *The Woodlanders,* where the fear of a tree falling on the house, prevented an old man from facing the reality of his life. When it was chopped down, he was forced to face it and died suddenly as a result.

Symptoms such as phobias and low self-esteem are the result of errors in storage of past experiences. You can use regression techniques to discover their origin, although desensitisation methods and suggestion, which are the most powerful means of dealing with these, do not require discovery of this. Only psychoanalytical methods would require that and, frankly, they don't have a very good cure record.

Self-punishment, or punishment of another

Self-punishment, or punishment of another person is often an unconscious cause of neurotic symptoms. The objective of therapy here is to bring about self-forgiveness, or forgiveness of the other person for a real or imagined past action. This is followed by verbalisation to bring about subconscious relearning.

If there is resistance to suggestion to forgive, regression, or parts therapy may be used to discover why. These methods will be explained shortly.

Discovering the symptom dynamic

One way to discover the symptom dynamic involved is to ask while your client is in trance. Here are some examples of the questions you might ask.

- Is this because of something that someone in authority has said to you in the past, which has had an enduring effect upon you?
- Is it due to your unconscious, dealing with a current unresolved issue?
- Is your unconscious causing this problem, because there is something else, which you are gaining as a result?
- Is it because you may be unconsciously identifying with someone else who behaves in this way?
- Are you unconsciously responding to an inner conflict, perhaps between two conflicting desires?
- Is the problem the result of some past event?
- Is it that you are unconsciously punishing yourself or someone else?

Ask these questions in a calm, monotonic voice, in order not to influence the response.

What if all, or most of the ideomotor responses are No, or Don't know ?

If all, or most of the ideomotor responses are *No* or *Don't know* this is not an ideal situation, but you can only work with the data you have. Many hypnotherapists hold the view that the way to enhance the value of this data is to treat the *Don't know* responses as potential Yes responses.

Advanced techniques for uncovering and releasing the problem

Affect bridge technique
The affect bridge method can be used as an effective uncovering technique. It works by using the emotions as a bridge between the present and the first time the problem was felt. The reasons it is useful for this is that, firstly, the emotions are the language of the unconscious, where the past event, its current effect and the cure are located. Secondly, unlike the analytical processes of the conscious mind, the emotions can transport the client's attention more or less instantaneously to the event.

Ask your client to imagine the problem and feel the emotions that go with it. Then regress them back to the onset of the problem. Suggest they feel it again and, this time, increase the intensity as you count from one to ten. You can also ask them to pinpoint where in the body they feel the effect. Here is an example:

One. Two. Three. Go deeper into that feeling now. ... Four, and five ... and as you feel it more and more intensely...going back further and further in time towards where it all started. Six. Seven ... stronger and more intense still... and it is so strong it is actually a relief to feel you are going back to where it all started. Eight. Nine.Ten.

Then snap your fingers and ask your client to be there and to report what is happening.

The drawback is that while it might take you to the first symptom-producing event, that may not be the same as the main sensitising event.

Dream analysis
Dream analysis under hypnosis is based on the premise that the unconscious speaks to us in dreams and the meaning becomes clear under hypnosis. With dream analysis, you may not need to induce a trance - just tell them to relive the dream and this will send them into a trance on its own.

When the client relates in the past tense, correct them, substituting with present tenses.

Don't automatically believe what the client says. There is always a danger of false memory syndrome. You need to examine, question and look for consistency and plausibility in their responses.

Regression to discover the onset of the problem.
Spontaneous regression
You may find that the client goes into a spontaneous regression. Unexpected emotional behaviour is a good indicator that this is

happening. For example, signs of emotional disturbance, discomfort, or even abreaction (emotional outpouring, usually with tears).

If this happens, it may be a good idea to calm it down, with suggestions that they should imagine viewing it as a film, or as a bystanding observer.

Allow the client to stay in this state for no more than sixty seconds, until the abreaction starts to subside. Guide them out of it with words such as:

Let the image fade now and go to your peaceful place. You can return to the issue and deal with it at a later time. Now just clear your mind and enjoy being in your own wonderful place of relaxation.

Ask your client if they are now ready to continue with the therapy. Repeat, if necessary, until an ideomotor response is given.

Ask them to imagine their desired outcome now. Don't suggest what *you* believe is happening. Remember, your client is very suggestible in a trance. They want to please the therapist, so don't make suggestions that will influence their perception. Use the six analytical questions - who, what, when, where, how and why - to fully explore the client's experience.

Hypnosis will not guarantee the truth comes out. Clients can still lie if they want to. The likelihood of this can be lessened by proper build-up of rapport, because it will increase the client's trust in you.

This is a protocol for regression:

- Establish client is in their own place of relaxation
- Establish ideomotor response signals
- Verify the depth of the trance
- Explain that in the trance there is only the present
- Assure your client of confidentiality
- Explain how false memory syndrome can occur through suggestion, deletions, distortions and generalisations. Point out that our emotions distort our perceptions of reality, but we respond to them as if they are undistorted.

The objective of this process is to reveal the perception that is causing the problem and then facilitate release and relearning

Your client must indicate their willingness to release the problem by ideomotor response (raising the *Yes* finger).

Verify the depth of trance

Verify the depth of trance by asking them to say how deep they are on a scale of 1 to 100, where 100 is as deeply as you can go in hypnosis and 50 is halfway there. Ask them to respond by raising the *Yes* and/or *No* fingers. Ask:

Are you 50 or deeper?

When you receive a *Yes* response, continue with deepening and then ask:

Are you 30 or deeper?

When you receive a *Yes* response, continue deepening further and then ask:

Are you deep enough to continue to the next stage?

If a client cannot get below 50, they are probably, highly analytical in their thinking style and even if they try to relive the problem experience, their analytical nature may well neutralise the emotionality of their images. If they don't go deep enough, then use the session to prepare them, by hypnotic suggestion, for a subsequent session.

If the client says they are 30 or below they are usually deep enough to accept suggestions to be regressed

The regression,

Here is an example of how to regress your client:

And now you drift...comfortably deeper... into a deep and pleasant state of relaxation. ... And you may already be aware...that you are drifting back in time....Stop me by raising your Yes finger when you get to an important year,...an important event that is related to the present problem.... And still drifting backwards to when you were 45,... and going even further back... 40, 35, 30... and back even further.

If your client previously told you when the problem was first experienced you can count backwards until you reach it, otherwise let your client guide you.

Continue as follows:

And now you can feel yourself getting younger

When you get to the teenage years, you can include suggestions like:

And you are aware that your limbs and your height are getting smaller in relation to adults around you.

If your client stops, watch and listen carefully. If they display emotional behaviour, command them to:

Report, what is happening now!"

Are you alone, or with others?

Who?

What can you see?

What do you feel?

What can you hear?

If they talk in the past tense, they are remembering rather than reliving.

You will recognise the significance of experiences in a report by the strength and nature of the emotional responses that accompany them. Remember, however, that it is not for you to pronounce that they are related to the cause of the problem, only to make the client aware of the recall experience and help them to make up their own mind about it.

Another way of regressing is by calendar years. The script is basically the same, except that, instead of ages, you use calendar years. Adults tend to remember past events by the year in which they occurred, perhaps better than the age they were at that time. One age is much like another in adulthood, but particular calendar years are memorable, because of events, fashions and music prevalent at the time.

Another means of age regression is to ask your client to go back to a happy time and place in childhood, but if they had an unhappy childhood this won't work.

10

Treating the problem

Maladaptation to past experiences

Many emotional problems are due to past experiences that have not been properly dealt with.

Disturbing experiences are a normal fact of life and, while they upset our mental well-being for a while, we normally come to terms with them in time. That time is dependent upon the severity of the trauma. An unkind putdown may make us feel hurt and damage our self-confidence for just a few hours, but a bereavement will cause grief for a year or so.

Sometimes, however, emotional trauma is too intolerable to a person's mind and emotions for them to even begin the healing process. In such cases, the person will deal with it in a maladaptive way.

If a person responds to trauma in a maladaptive way they do not come to terms with it. The experience continues to have its raw, traumatic effect. The emotional and behavioural outcomes, however, may not appear to be related to the trauma. Such maladaptations are often the causes of neurotic symptoms that a client may present to a hypnotherapist. Typical types of Maladaptation are as follows:

- Denial
- Displacement
- Identification
- Rationalisation
- Reaction formation
- Repression
- Reversal

Maladaptation and neurotic symptoms

Anxiety is the basic substance of neurotic symptoms, but there may also be things like depression, low self-esteem, phobias, troublesome internal dialogues, or panic attacks, to name just a few of the other symptoms that may be present.

Clinical depression

One of the ways that these maladaptations can result in clinical depression is as a result of reversal - the turning of antipathy towards another person inwards upon themselves.

Types of anxiety

Anxiety can be analysed into four easily identifiable types:

- Free-floating anxiety.
- Neurotic anxiety
- Moral anxiety
- Existential anxiety

Free-floating anxiety is where a person feels generally anxious for no apparent reason. Neurotic anxiety causes a person to fear they may overstep the moral boundaries. Moral anxiety is where a person fears their moral concerns will overly limit their ability to behave normally. Existential anxiety derives from feelings of insecurity as a result of a person's acute awareness of their own existence. Often they are relatively preoccupied with the existential questions of why they exist and just what it means to exist.

Maladaptations can produce their emotional effect in any of these anxiety forms. Free-floating anxiety is the root, or primary form of which the other forms are species. The former is the most difficult to deal with, as it has no object, or focus and so offers no immediate hope of relief. This is why it often anchors itself onto an obsessive and unwarranted concern and becomes one of the derivative species. These are easier to deal with moment by moment, but are more debilitating in the long run.

Developmental maladaptations

Failure to make adaptive responses during the developmental stages of life can stunt a person's mental maturity and leave unresolved developmental business in the emotional sphere. This causes a variety of problems in adult life.

Unresolved Oedipus and Electra complexes are typical examples. The Oedipus complex is the stage of life where, according to Freudian theory, a male child, in fear of his father, turns away from his, hitherto, predominant orientation towards his mother. Instead, he orientates towards his father, upon whom he then models his own behaviour. The Electra complex is the female version of the Oedipus complex and works roughly in the opposite way.

At a later stage, in puberty, the male adolescent confronts and stands up to his father, thereby developing an autonomous adult self and vice versa with a female. If a father is so aggressive, or an adolescent so sensitive that this does not fully take place the developmental stage remains incomplete. This is believed, by adherents of psychoanalysis, to cause a wide variety of neurotic symptoms.

Phobias
Phobias can be caused several different ways:

- Classical conditioning.
- Operant conditioning
- Social modelling
- Projection

Classical conditioning
By far the most prevalent cause of phobias is classical conditioning. When two things are perceived within fifteen seconds of each other, one an event and the other an emotion, the unconscious associates them, so that when such an event occurs again the same emotion will be triggered.

Phobic fear of spiders (arachnophobia) becomes established when a child is suddenly frightened (perhaps by the sound of their parents rowing, or the sound of thunder, or whatever) and, within 15 seconds, it picks up, in its peripheral vision, a spider, somewhere on the wall. There are frequently spiders somewhere within our peripheral vision; we just don't always perceive them consciously. The unconscious doesn't miss them, though. The latter takes in a great deal more data than the conscious, and it stores such associations. Whenever a spider is seen thereafter it triggers the fear emotion. Each time this occurs the strength of the fear may be increased.

Operant conditioning
Operant conditioning refers to a process whereby a person witnesses another person gaining an emotional reward for displaying a particular behaviour. Arachnophobia and various other phobias can arise in this way, where a sibling displays fear of an object and receives the comforting attention of their mother for doing so. The other sibling learns, unconsciously, that such a display of fear is associated with maternal, or other comforting attention.

Social modelling
Social modelling refers to the way some phobias simply develop as a result of a child modelling their own behaviour on that of another person. Everybody copies models as they develop into adulthood and some adults continue to do so thereafter. If the modelled behavioural

repertoire includes phobia or other neurotic symptoms then that may be included too.

Projection
Projection refers to a process whereby all the negative and unpalatable qualities of a person's self, or someone close to them is projected onto some other organism. A spider is an ideal candidate, because of its hideous appearance.

Any of these processes may underlie the symptoms with which a client presents to a hypnotherapist. The latter must try to discover which one, or more, of them it is.

Treating maladaptations
Traumas that have not been resolved by emotional and cognitive adaption need to be uncovered, relived and an appropriate adaption facilitated. This will often require an abreaction - an emotional outpouring, usually with tears.

Therapeutic abreaction
Abreactions, which can be due to real, or imagined events, can be therapeutic, as they can put a person back in touch with their emotions, with which they may have been out of touch for a long time. If an abreaction takes place when an underlying trauma is uncovered, then it is necessary and appropriate, for it wouldn't happen if there was not a dammed up well of pain.

If the abreaction is thought to be too strong and painful, instruct the client to let it fade away. Say:

Now clear your mind... go deeply back into your comfortable state of relaxation.

After a while, take the client back to the time of the trauma, but suggest to them that it will not be so strong this time and get their consent and confirmation of willingness to return to it.

An alternative way of watering down the experience is to instruct them to visit the scene as an observer, or to imagine they are seeing it on a film screen. This puts a bit of emotional space between the client and the trauma and allows them to adapt to it gradually.

Revivification
You need to ensure that the client is not just remembering the event, rather than reliving it. You can achieve this by asking them questions in the present tense and correcting them every time they use the past tense in their responses. If they persist in using the past tense, deepen the induction.

The empty chair method

The empty chair method is a process by which a person can project all the feelings they have bottled up towards another person - a parent, a partner, a sibling, a friend, or an authority figure onto an empty chair in which they visualise the correct object of those feelings. This facilitates appropriate adaption, because   of the mind/body consistency that has been well proven to prevail in humans. If you behave as if something is the case your mind will respond as if that is the case and vice versa.

If circumstances prevent this consistency anxiety results. Lying and the consequent guilt that follows is a simple example of this.

So the objective is to get the client to re-enact a situation where, in the past, they did not respond as they ought to have done - spoke their mind, stood up to an oppressor, or whatever. Thus, their mind will be relieved as a result of doing what it ought to have done a long while ago.

Acting something out has the same effect on the emotions as if the situation was real, although not quite as intense. Indeed, actors become quite traumatised by emotional scenes and their real characters develop in a way that follows naturally from the behaviours of those characters they play on stage and screen. As a result, they tend to develop very complex and multiple personalities. Sometimes, as a result, it is difficult to perceive quite what is their real self.

This method is particularly appropriate where symptoms are due to an unresolved developmental crisis, such as the Oedipus, or Electra complex.

The empty chair method can also facilitate the situation where a client can forgive and let go. A variation of this is where the clients are invited to sit in the empty chair themselves and respond to their own statements. This will   facilitate an understanding of the other's point of view. If they can't forgive them understanding is the next best thing. Grudges have to be dispensed with, as full emotional release cannot be achieved otherwise.

After the treatment, bring the client back to their place of relaxation and ask them to verbalise the new insights they have gained. Ask what they have learned that will be of benefit to them.

Insights that are verbalised under hypnosis are particularly powerful, because of the heightened state of suggestibility that the client is in when they do so. It is in this way that powerful relearning is achieved.

Systematic desensitisation

Systematic desensitisation is a useful method of correcting for phobias. It does not remove the phobia, it just overlays the maladaptive pair of perceptions stored in the unconscious with a more appropriate stored pair - the spider and something pleasant, instead of the spider and something fearful.

The process is carried out gradually, using diluted versions of the stimulus, gradually increasing in realism, until they equal the real phobic object. For example, an arachnophobic client might be shown a cartoon picture of a lovable spider at the same time as experiencing a positive emotion brought about by suggestion under trance conditions. Subsequently, perhaps, a plastic spider might be used, then a real money-spider and so on, until the client can actually touch the leg of a full-sized house spider without paralysing fear.

After the desensitisation session, the client should be taken back to their place of relaxation and asked to verbalise their new insights, which, under the influence of hypnosis, will have a powerful, and enduring effect, for reasons already mentioned. The new adaption will last as long as they do not have another strongly, traumatic spider experience. If they do the old, paired data will become dominant again and the phobia will return. However, it can be treated again and again by the same techniques, so it is manageable.

Treating Addictions

Addictions are conditions that persist because of the fact that they offer a false reward. They offer very short-term relief from anxiety, but in the longer term, they cause it to increase, along with a whole host of other problems, the most serious of which are related to health.

The short-term rewards that these habits offer are never simple and, on the contrary, are often multiplex.

Smoking addiction

In the case of smoking, for example, the rewards are:

- Chemical (nicotine)
- Social (conforming to the norms of the group)
- Satisfaction of conditioned habit (smoking follows a meal, etc.)
- Distraction from social anxiety (focus on the cigarette instead of the people present)
- Relief from worry (focus on the cigarette instead of the problem), providing something to do with your hands

and so on.

False reasoning

Any reasonably intelligent person knows that it is a very unwise thing to do, but the combination of the many strands of relief that keep the addiction going are so powerful that they overwhelm the strength of the addict's will to resist them. The conflict causes their own conscious mind to trick them into false reasoning. Examples are beliefs that:

- they have broken the habit and now they can keep their smoking to a safe level.

- they could get knocked down by a bus and killed, in which case struggling to quit smoking beforehand would have been a waste of time.

- there will be plenty of time to quit later.

The addiction-hijacked consciousness creates no end of arguments for continuing with addictive behaviour, whatever kind of addiction it is.

Will strengthening
As these addictions are due to a relative weakness of the will, in comparison to the addiction forces, the only way of correcting for this weakness is to strengthen the will, so that it wins the battle. Hypnotherapy is in its element where strengthening of the will is concerned.

Glove anaesthesia for pain management.
Glove anaesthesia is a technique that involves getting a client to imagine numbness you have induced in their hand is being transferred to an area of pain in their body, which they touch.
Talk with the client about exploring the power of the mind. Obtain permission to touch them.

Induce arm catalepsy and ideomotor response.
Ask the client to imagine that there is a bucket of ice in front of them. You can enhance the suggestion with a description of the kind of bucket in which champagne might be served. You can even have such a bucket of ice handy, so that you can invoke the sound of ice chinking in it. Don't let the client put their hand into it, though. It's only there for sound effects.
   Tell them to imagine they are placing a cataleptic arm into the bucket, right up to the wrist. Aid the client's imagination, by suggesting that their hand is getting colder and colder, more and more numb, and then suggest that there is a complete absence of any feeling in their hand.

Tell the client that in a moment you will awaken them and even though they are fully awake, the complete numbness in their hand will remain. Count from one to three and ask the client to open their eyes. Test their hand for sensation, by pinching with gradually increasing pressure.

Now induce a deep trance and install an ideomotor response, i.e ask your client to designate a *yes, no* and *don't know* finger.

Place the client's hand into the area of pain and make the following suggestion:

And as I count from 1 to 3... all of the numbness you feeling in that hand will spread into the area of pain and discomfort that you have been feeling ...and as it does...experiencing all that pain and discomfort gradually fading to an appropriate level.

Give your client a few minutes to explore this and then say:

When an appropriate level of numbness has been reached I want you to signal with your Yes finger.

Hypno-aversion therapy.

Hypno-aversion therapy is useful for treating persistent, unwanted habits. It involves deliberately inducing a phobia to the habit the client wants to get rid of.

First, you have to decide on a sufficiently aversive stimulus to use. It could be mouldy food, slime, bad eggs, stink bombs, or a variety of other aversive stimuli. Use your imagination. Anything the client reports as the most aversive stimulus they can imagine will be appropriate, as long as you can obtain it. There are some things that are repulsive to most, if not everybody, but some things will be more repulsive than others to particular people. This is your challenge in the gathering of therapy resources stage of this treatment. You need to enquire what is the most aversive stimulus that your client can imagine.

It is advisable to have a bowl and tissues to hand, in case the client actually vomits.

Making powerful suggestions

In general, the substance of your treatment of a client's condition is making suggestions to them while they are in a deeply relaxed and, therefore, receptive state. This is a state where their unconscious, analytical mind has been, to a large degree, neutralised by tricking their body into perceiving that its attention is not needed, or by keeping it occupied on other things. In this state, the suggestions will be accepted relatively uncritically, just as those that were made to them by authority figures, such as parents, when they were at an infantile age, before their conscious, analytical faculties were developed.

Uncovering the source errors of storage

If you are trying to correct a client's maladaptive behaviour in response to a stimulus, such as an exam situation, a public speaking engagement, a spider, an imminent aeroplane journey, crowds or whatever, then you need to uncover the errors of data storage in the client's mind that have given rise to the maladaptive complex. A person responds to stimuli at five different stages, each on a different level of mental processing.

1. Perception,
2. Matching with the memory matrix
3. Evaluation of what the stimulus means by recalling beliefs about it
4. Choosing the behavioural response
5. Evaluating whether it was the right one and how effective it was

Aim suggestions at as many matrix levels as are appropriate

Your suggestions, should deal with as many levels as are appropriate. For example, in suggesting that their perception was at error, if it was (and 80% of perception is guesswork), explain how and why it was in error.

Secondly, explain that the data they had stored in their memory matrix relating to this kind of stimulus is at error, for example in the case of a fear of flying, explain that it is not correct that flying is dangerous. You're far more likely to be killed in a car as in a plane, even if you spend the same amount of time in each.

Much flying phobia is due to a failure to understand how such a heavy thing as an aeroplane can stay in the sky. Gen yourself up and explain to them how aerofoils work. It's not about surfing the air, as many think. When they understand it, they should adjust their memory matrix. so that it doesn't rank as a dangerous exercise.

Make a suggestion aimed at the choice of behavioural response stage also. Tell them that now that they understand that it is not dangerous, there is no need to produce a fear response and that the best response is to keep themselves occupied by reading or talking, as this engages the conscious, analytical mind. When this is active the emotional unconscious is not in charge.

Strategically implanted suggestions in a *Quit smoking* session

To give you an example of how much detail and strategically placed suggestions you can use, let's again use the example of a *Quit smoking session,* as this is quite a common reason why someone will visit a hypnotherapist.

You have to change their perception that particular times and events are appropriate for having a cigarette. There is no reason to have a cigarette after a meal, at the end of a working day, when you have a drink, or when someone else's smoking. This is hypnotic suggestion at level 2.

Tell them they have a mind of their own and can decide for themselves that it is not necessary or appropriate. This is hypnotic suggestion at level 3.

Changing the data they have stored

You need to make suggestions to change the data they have stored on the practice of smoking – from perceiving it as an acceptable, social habit to perceiving it as a dangerous, antisocial habit.

You need also to correct their understanding of the health risks involved. Spend some time on this. Educate them, also, on how the narcotic effects distort the perception and understanding of the appropriateness and the risks of smoking.

Following this, you need to make suggestions about how they will respond behaviourally to the urges to smoke and the usual environmental cues that trigger such behaviour in the future.

Use all the modalities and sub modalities

When you're making the suggestions, you need to make the memories stick. You can do this by being very descriptive in all of the modalities - visual, kinaesthetic, auditory, olfactory and gustatory and the sub-modalities of these, including colours, shapes and sizes, hard/soft, texture, large/small, high/low, fragrant, stale, pleasant/unpleasant, sweet, savoury, bitter, sour, etc.[26,27]

Dealing with the narcotic self-deception

Say to your entranced client:

One of the big mistakes that quitters make is, after a while, thinking to themselves that they have kicked the habit, so just having one cigarette won't harm. This is only the narcotics tricking their mind, in

---

[26] Marshall (2012c) Ch.4
[27] Marshall (2012f) Ch.2

a desperate attempt to keep the habit going. It's amazing how the unconscious works – It thinks you need the nicotine and will trick you, if it has to, in order to get it. But you won't yield to it. Your will is too strong. You will see such feelings for what they really are and won't be fooled by them. All addictions involve self-deception and people who quit and start again tend to smoke even more. If you feel the pangs of withdrawal embrace them as a bodybuilder embraces muscle pain. Think - No pain, no gain!

Grim data you want to implant

Here is an example of the kind of script you can use to implant the grim facts.

Smoking is antisocial, as it creates bad breath. ... It's extremely costly. ...Smokers' fingers are always stained with nicotine and their teeth become stained. ...Smoking causes lung cancer, stomach and other cancers. ...It is a class A carcinogen. ... It causes heart disease, arteriosclerosis and stroke. ... It causes emphysema and premature skin ageing. ... It kills vitamins ... and impairs oxygen intake, which is necessary for tissue repair. There are 97,000 smoking-related deaths per year in the UK. ... One in five of all deaths is due to smoking. ... This is the because there are more than 4000 chemicals in cigarette smoke. ... Smoking kills four times as many people as all the other known causes put together. ... See the immensity of the risk? ... Imagine a game of Russian roulette ... each of three people spins the gun in the centre and whoever it points to fires it at their neighbour. ... Would you play it? ... No, of course you wouldn't, even if you were offered millions of pounds ... but understand this very clearly! ... You would have more chance of dying eventually from smoking ... as you would immediately from that cause. ... Smoking will kill one out of every two people who smoke. ... You would have more chance of staying alive than if you continue to smoke ... for the game of Russian Roulette would kill one in three ... while smoking will strike down one in two who continue to smoke. ... That is a hard ... abundantly proven ... fact. ... Smoking is more deadly than Russian Roulette.
Why don't people take notice of it? ... Because it's too horrible. ... 97,000 smoking-related deaths a year. ... There are more than 4000 harmful chemicals in cigarette smoke ... including benzene - one of the most cancer-causing substances known to us ... formaldehyde - you see the hazard signs on lorries carrying the stuff. ... Other chemicals include ammonia ... cyanide, ... acetone ... arsenic ... nicotine and carbon monoxide. The latter is the chemical some suicides choose ... Carbon monoxide is a poisonous gas that binds to haemoglobin, the carrier of oxygen carrier to other parts of the body.

... Fifteen percent of the blood of smokers is carrying carbon monoxide instead of oxygen.

Here are some facts for you to face up to: ... The average smoker dies 10 to 15 years earlier than they would if they didn't smoke. Young men are 42 times more likely to die of smoking-related diseases than of being killed on the road. ... Women who smoke run a greater risk of miscarriage or giving premature birth. Tobacco addicts deceive themselves with excuses such as 'The damage is done now; it's too late.' ... But if you stop smoking before you get heart disease or lung cancer you will avoid nearly all the risks of premature death. Self-deceiving clients say, 'I could get run over by a bus, so the struggle to quit would be a waste of time. ... However, this, too, is typical of the way the narcotics in tobacco trick the mind to keep the habit going. ... The truth is, as you know ... you almost certainly won't be run over by a bus or anything else. ... Very few people are. ... but smoking damages every smoker's health ... and most will die before their time.

Making suggestions at the response level
This is how you could input your response level suggestions:

Your daily routine is a map of cues for triggering your smoking habit ... so you will change your routine to avoid where the smoking cues are placed. ... After a meal, for example ... you will get straight up from the table, rather than continuing to sit there. When you feel a pang of withdrawal ... or the urge for a cigarette ... you will do something else to occupy yourself, ... such as plan what to do with the money you are saving ... and the effect will pass. You will regularly look into the mirror and say to yourself ... 'I am a non-smoker'... The cognitive dissonance effect that binds the actions of mind and body together will cause your natural inclinations ... to become more and more consistent with your words. You will become increasingly inclined ... to be a non-smoker. Quitting may seem a little difficult at first ... but every day it will get easier. ... You'll have more energy. ... Therefore, you must do something with it. Smokers feel being a smoker is part of their identity ... but you must face the fact that the real nature of addiction ... is not part of your identity. By quitting smoking, you will think more clearly. ... You'll be more alert. ... You will look more confident. ... It is not part of you.

Choice of treatment method
You will have already decided on the method of treatment you are going to use. It will depend on both the type of problem the client has and the discipline you prefer and in which you have trained.

If you are from a behaviourist psychology background, you may well favour conditioning methods, such as systematic desensitisation.

If you identify yourself with the psychoanalytical school you may rely on regression and catharsis. If you believe that cognitive psychology is the best way of treating neurotic conditions you are likely to rely on revealing the errors in the client's thinking that are causing the problem and train them to think in more constructive and appropriate ways.

Whichever of these treatment approaches you use, you will be using hypnosis to augment your psychotherapy, by making the client more receptive to the treatment.

If your client has come to you for self-improvement purposes, rather than to treat any malady, you will be using hypnosis for ego strengthening and/or installation of a post hypnotic cue or cues.

There is another way, however, that hypnosis can be used in therapy and this is perhaps the most interesting and relevant of all. It is to this that I turn next.

The trance explanation of neurotic symptoms

There is an approach that is unique to hypnotherapy and which provides a very plausible explanation of all neurotic symptoms. These are symptoms caused by experiences, rather than neuro-chemical imbalances in the brain, wiring faults, genetic factors, or damage from illness or trauma.

This approach provides that all neurotic illnesses are caused by trance phenomena in the past. The neurotic symptoms arise when, unwittingly, a person's self-hypnotises and implants troublesome posthypnotic suggestions. The way to resolve the error is for a professional hypnotist to re-hypnotise them and implant other, more appropriate and more powerful ones.

This may sound odd at first, but when you look at it in detail, it makes sense and is not inconsistent with any other school of thought.

What is a trance?

A trance is a situation where a person is completely absorbed in something to the exclusion of everything else. We all spend a fair percentage of our time in trance, for example, when we read a book, watch a film, build a model, write a letter, or just daydream.

Trance phenomena

What makes a trance different from a non-trance state is that trance phenomena are present. Trance phenomena (referred to by professionals as TP) includes:

- Positive hallucination
- Negative hallucination

- Age progression.
- Age regression.
- Time distortion.
- Sensory distortion
- Dissociation
- Amnesia
- Posthypnotic suggestions

Hallucinations

Positive hallucinations
A hallucination is an experience that is felt, to some degree, as real. When we read a book, watch a film, or daydream we, to some degree, suspend belief that the experience is not real. If we didn't we would not feel the emotions of the experience.

Negative hallucinations
Negative hallucinations are fears that are felt as result of anticipating that something won't happen.

Age progression and regression
When we daydream about what we will do at some future time we are progressing our age forward and when we reminisce on the past we are regressing it. It is not that we are simply remembering it. If that were so we would not feel the emotions connected with the experience. The fact that we do is evidence that we are reliving it to some degree and if we are reliving it we must have mentally regressed our age.

Time distortion
You will, no doubt, have noticed that a good film seems to whizz through quickly while a boring film drags. This is because you are more fully absorbed in a gripping film and you experience time distortion.

How many people can say they have not known a situation where they have been deep in thought, suddenly realised that they have missed their exit from the motorway and travelled on miles further than they should have done. This is another example of time distortion in trance.

Sensory distortion
When a person is worried about a pain the pain becomes more noticeable and often gets worse. Sometimes the pain only occurs after the worry starts. When that person becomes absorbed in something

else, so that they don't think about the pain, often it will disappear. This is an example of the sensory distortion that characterises trances.

When a person is in a trance, whether because they are watching a film or listening to an interesting story, everything else in their perceptual field is blocked out. This is what conjurers rely on. They absorb the audience's attention so that they miss everything else that is occurring around the focus of the trick.

Dissociation

Dissociation occurs when a person does not feel any of the normal emotional feelings that ought to result from an experience. They do this by unwittingly entering an unrelated trance that taps their emotions. This is commonly found where a newly bereaved person can only think of some unrelated concern, such as whether they remembered to switch the cooker off before they left the house.

Amnesia

Amnesia refers to an inability to remember things. There are two basic categories - *anterograde* and *retrograde* amnesia. We are only concerned with the latter here, as the other concept refers to a physical brain fault that prevents a person making new memories. Hypnotherapy can't help with that one. Retrograde amnesia, which it often can help with, has several types.

- Dissociative fugue - a general inability to recall things from before a specific point in time,
- Lacunar amnesia - an inability to recall a specific event
- Childhood amnesia - an inability to recall events from childhood.

Posthypnotic suggestions.

Everyone has experienced how a particular smell can rapidly transport their attention back in time to a previous experience, and they suddenly feel all the emotions connected with it. All the associated sensory phenomena are re-experienced too - the sights, the sounds, the smells, the tastes and the physical sensations. This is because these events or circumstances were originally experienced in a highly absorbing way that blocked out all extraneous things, creating tunnel vision and a powerful, multisensory channel experience.

Those were the ideal conditions for the sensory phenomena to give rise to posthypnotic suggestions. The different elements of the experience will have been stored in such a way that the unconscious would interpret the combination as a suggestion that they are inseparably connected.

How these trance phenomena alone can result in future neuroses
In the future, if any one these phenomena are encountered the whole complex of them will be felt. Just as pleasurable emotions can be projected forward in this way so can troubling ones. These can
produce future feelings of fear, guilt, shame, insecurity, grief, anxiety, and so on. The list covers every kind of neurotic symptom that a hypnotherapist will encounter.

When clients present themselves and explain the symptoms they are already in the trance. The task of the hypnotist is to hypnotise them and get them out of the trance that is causing the problem.

Problematic trance states
A problematic trance state exists when an event produces a response that we cannot control or get out of. It is the presence of choice of responses that determines whether the trance becomes a problematic one. When we have no range of responses and, therefore, no control, we fall into a trance, where our response is controlled by the unconscious.

This is why installing an alternative response, or perception, or evaluation works, because it gives the client an alternative response and, therefore, some control. The job of the therapist is to interpret and delete negative trance states, or give the client a chance to exit them.

Characteristics of trance states
Wolinski [28] identified three core characteristics of trance states:

- Tunnel vision
- Usually experienced as something that is happening to the person
- Spontaneous emergence of trance phenomena

Trance states also:
- have a beginning, middle and end
- are manipulable processes
- feature a cluster of trance phenomena

Trance states are created in childhood, whenever a child's ability to handle an experience has been exceeded. The problem is that trances created early in infancy may have served a useful purpose at that

---

[28] Wolinski (2007)

stage of life, in a particular instance, but it is then generalised to all similar situations in subsequent life and will not be appropriate, or useful then. Moreover, these trance states may be problematic and cause the symptoms that the client presents to the therapist.

The hypnotherapist's remedy

The remedy is to hypnotise the client and put things right. You can't actually erase what has been implanted, because the implantation is memory storage and this involves structural changes in the brain circuitry. You can't undo these changes by suggestion. What you can do, however, is implant a suggestion that will be more powerful than the troubling one and which will contradict it.

You will have noticed the similarity between this explanation and remedy and those that the behaviourist therapists use (see p.89.). The difference is that, to the latter, the maladaptive storage occurs purely because of the degree of contiguity of stimulus and response, i.e. the time span within which the connected events or circumstances on the one hand and the emotional feelings on the other occur. Fifteen to thirty seconds is the crucial parameter. The trance explanation, however, provides that it is the intensity of the stimuli and the receptiveness of the individual's immature mind at the time that is the catalyst. It would be naïve for the hypnotherapist to dispute the contiguity effect, because it is well proven but, likewise, the behaviourists would be naïve to dispute the effect of trance. It is reasonable to conclude that both are contributory factors.

Where do we start, then? First, we need to fully understand the mechanism by which the troublesome data was stored, so that we can target our suggestions to the right parts of the system – the bits that need counteracting with new, contradictory data. A model that reveals to us the whole, multiplex storage system is known as the matrix model.

In fact, whichever approach to treatment you use, it is very important to target your suggestions right, as otherwise they will be ineffective. To understand how and where to target them, we need to study the complex processes that the human mind goes through in the chain from stimulus to response.

You may decide you need to aim your suggestions at one part, several parts, or at every part of the matrix. The rationale for the latter is the mudslinging effect. Throw enough of it and some of it is likely to land in the right place.

The matrix model

The matrix model maps out the steps that the mind makes in storing and responding to a situation. They are as follows:

- Stimulus
- Emotion
- Response
- Termination
- evaluation

While our unconscious processes about 2 million bits of sensory data per second, our conscious mind is aware of only 7 ± 2 bits. This means that an awful lot of selection is going on. It also means that almost everything is missed by the consciousness, but not by the unconscious.

How the selection is done

The way the conscious selects the data to perceive is on the basis of that which presents itself as the most powerful and the most relevant to survival and that which comes in the form of the data modalities towards which the person's system is biased. For example , some people are particularly visual; others are more auditory, olfactory, gustatory or kinaesthetic

The small amount of data that is selected by the thalamus is directed to the various parts of the brain that specialise in processing data of that modality and sub modality. Sub modalities of the visual sense include, for example: scale, colour, brightness, etc. Those of the auditory sense include such things as amplitude, pitch, tone, etc. Sub modalities of the gustatory modality include: sweet, sour, bitter, savoury, and so on. Those of the olfactory sense include the range of smells available to human perception and the sub modalities of the kinesthetic modality include anything felt physically in the body, including joy, sadness, grief, fear, pain, aches, tickles, warmth, cold and so on.

The clearest memories are those that are coded in the most modalities and sub modalities[29,30].

All in the mind

After this process, the information arrives back at the thalamus elaborated with 80% more data from previously stored and processed information, so most of what arrives back in the thalamus as perception has not come from the environment at all, but from the person's own mind. It makes the saying *all in the mind* very relevant. It is, therefore, easy to see how our stored sensory data can be inappropriate and troublesome in the future.

---

[29] Marshall (2012c) pp.40-43.
[30] Marshall (2012f) Ch.2.

How the data is reduced to 7± 2 bits.

We know how the data is selected and reduced in the process of perception. There are three principal mechanisms:

- Deletion
- Distortion
- Generalisation

Deletion

Deletion is one part of the process by which the conscious deletes from its perception everything except 7±2 bits of data that satisfy the criteria already mentioned.

The more something is seen, the less it is noticed. This is called recurrent inhibition. When the same phenomena are encountered day after day, they are unlikely to be threatening to the individual. It's only when things are different that they may pose a threat, so the perceptual mechanism, limited as it is, has adapted to spot only the things that appear different[31].

Distortion

The perceptual process looks for quick matches with stored images and ignores any slight differences. The level of difference at which the conscious mind identifies something as different to what it has stored is known as the difference threshold.

Generalisation

Generalisation takes place by means of three mental algorithms:

- Cause and effect $A \rightarrow B$
- Complex equivalence $A = B$
- Difference $A \neq B$

Very often it is bad generalisations made by the unconscious that have caused the problem.

Further distortion of the data

Stored feelings from the past are relived before the related events are recalled, that is if the latter can be recalled at all. Many of the events, or circumstances that originally gave rise to the stored, emotional responses will have been wholly, or partly deleted, or repressed. In fact, this will usually be the case when the events were traumatic.

---

[31] Marshall (2012) Ch. 3.

Even to the extent that they have not, they will have been distorted in the storage process for reasons already explained. After feelings have been relived, the need to remain in executive control will make a person rationalises those feelings and this may distort the accuracy of the memories that gave rise to them. Moreover, each time this happens it will distort them even more.

When emotional responses are re-experienced the unconscious automatically regards the response that it stored as appropriate – even if was an inappropriate one.

Five levels of mental operation

Bateson[32] proposed that five levels of operation explain how the brain and body's resources combine to formulate and execute responses and interpret, modify and store the memories of events. This model provides that our identity determines our values and beliefs. These, in turn, organise our capabilities, which are due to the mental maps and strategies we hold and determine the way we will respond to stimuli within whatever external constraints prevail.

- the environmental stimulus.
- the client's relevant beliefs and values
- their capabilities to deal with the stimulus
- their behavioural repertoire
- their identity

Five levels of mental operation

Non-trance and trance identities

Human beings have a tendency to develop trance identities. When we are being controlled by strong emotion, we are in a trance identity that is controlling our behaviour. The emergence of the trance identity will usually be triggered by environmental phenomena.

Trance identities have the same five levels of operation as non-trance identities, all of which support their persistence. Each trance identity has its own matrix and this creates particular beliefs and personal values about what is important and relevant. These in turn will determine an individual's responses.

---

[32] Bateson, (1972) Steps to an Ecology of Mind London: Paladin, Granada

Capabilities in trance identities tend to be limited. The beliefs belonging to particular trance identities lead to unconscious inevitabilities about our behavioural tendencies, emotional outcomes and lifestyle, inevitabilities.

Emotional hijacking

This is how a problematic trance identity forms in childhood. Our conscious mind (the ego) interprets events and circumstances and chooses the emotions we should feel in response to them. If the initial emotion is felt too strongly, however, the ego will become overwhelmed, give up and hide, leaving the amygdala in charge. This tiny, almond-shaped part of the brain knows only one kind of emotion – fear. It is the fear centre of the brain and it has no rationality. It functions chaotically. The emotions surge and fear runs riot. Such a situation is commonly referred to by therapists as emotional hijacking and the trigger event is referred to as a *SEE*, standing for *significant emotional event*.

When an emotional hijacking has taken place the conscious intelligence has lost control and the person is in a trance and in the trance state, evolutionary responses rule. These are largely limited to the use of nominal processing. The trance will continue until the situation is no longer present. Then, the parasympathetic nervous system will release endorphins, calm the person and normal cognitive functioning will return.

The parasympathetic nervous system will also activate in situations of nervous exhaustion. The latter will eventually result from prolonged emotional hijacking.

The range of emotions and modes of processing

Before we go further, we need to look at the range of emotions and the kinds of processing available to the perceptual system. Let's deal with emotions first. The range can be split into two distinct categories, primary emotions and process emotions. Primary emotions are innate and relate to physical survival. There are three of them that are relevant here:

- Fear
- Anger
- Pleasure

Process emotions are combinations of these that produce more finely tuned feelings. These develop as an individual matures and interacts with their environment. They relate to social survival rather than physical survival. They are feelings about ourselves, how okay we are and the rules we hold about the behaviour of ourselves and others.

No matter how old, or mature a person is, if their physical survival is threatened primary emotions will rule. Loss of a partner, for example, can make survival so difficult that primary emotions take over. Our unconscious functions to protect us, producing what it thinks are relevant emotional and physical responses.

Modes of processing

Just as the range of emotions available change as we mature and develop the modes of processing available to the perceptual faculties also change. The range of processing modes is as follows.

- Nominal
- Ordinal
- Interval
- Ratio

Nominal processing

Nominal processing refers to the manner in which an infant processes information about the world. There is no relating or comparison between one thing and another. Everything it experiences is a stimulus completely in its own right. A thing, or an experience is either frightening, or annoying, or pleasurable, rather than being a bit more, or a bit less frightening or pleasurable than something else.

Ordinal processing

Ordinal processing is more sophisticated and develops later in childhood. Here things are ordered so that, for example, any adult's smiling face is perceived as pleasurable, the face of a familiar person is even more so and the sight of their mother's face is even more pleasurable still.

Interval processing

Interval processing is even more sophisticated. This kind of processing gauges the difference between one thing and another.

Ratio processing

Ratio processing is even more sophisticated still. It involves comparing the proportions of one thing with another.

Consequently, these different levels of sophistication in processing experiential data involve different levels of sophistication in choice of emotional response.

Problems start in infancy

Given that infants have no sophistication in their manner of processing, - something is either frightening or it is not; there are no shades of grey - it is not surprising that SEEs, where the ego abdicates power in favour of the amygdala, are more likely in this stage of life.

Most neurotic symptoms date back to childhood, when the matrix matching ability is not yet fully mature and where nominal processing occurred.

As the modes of processing change, as the child matures, the fear objects become related and compared to similar objects and experiences and the potentials of each compared. This results in generalisation of the phobic response. Similar objects to the phobic object become fear- inducing to a lesser extent according to their similarity to the primary phobic object.

Responses become increasingly inappropriate

Nor is it surprising that the original experience becomes lost in the memory, leaving only the troubling emotional response, because as the child matures and develops gradually into adulthood. so it's modes of processing change, so that each time it recalls the experience it interprets it differently and re-stores it changed as a result. By adulthood, the memory will be significantly different to the original experience. Indeed, the latter may no longer even be remembered.

This is why stored early perceptions that influence our response to situations in adult life are often so inappropriate. If we had been adults when we first had these experiences we would respond to them very differently.

Small changes are generative

Redefinition of past events will change current responses to them and these will continue to change over time. Furthermore, small initial changes increasing lead to major distortion of the memories, because of what is known as the butterfly effect. Such changes can be anywhere and everywhere in the matrix.

The Butterfly effect explains why an SEE can be trivial compared with its future consequences and why people often report that consequences become more noticeable over time. Adding to this, older people have a more developed, master matrix, so maladaptations will be more persistent.

Evaluation

The unconscious mind appraises how successfully the matrix strategy for solving the problem has been in protecting the emotional well-being of the person.

This evaluation phase is very important in therapy and, as a hypnotherapist, you can influence the outcome. Direct your client, both consciously and while in trance, to notice anything about their response that was different to what they expected. Not only does this reinforce the changes in their model of the world, but getting your client to notice the changes activates the left-brain function of logic and rational thinking.

There will also be interval and ratio processing involved, where the previous state of the matrix was based on only nominal and more primitive forms of analysis in childhood, when the initial traces were laid down. In the evaluation process, by directing the client to focus on what is different to what it used to be, they will also tend to focus on what was once background information, rather than what was in the focal view.

This conscious convincing will lead to unconscious change in the matrix.

Changing the matrix

As long as the original event or circumstances have not been deleted, then the trick is to reproduce the original event and encourage a more adaptive response for the client's matrix to hold. If the original event or circumstances have been repressed, but not deleted they should be able to be retrieved under hypnosis.

Regressive techniques can be useful for discovering the initial SEE, so that it can be reinterpreted constructively with the aid of the therapist. The matrix will be modified as a result and when accessed to match the same experiential data in the future it will no longer invoke the same emotional response. The basic purpose of all post-hypnotic suggestions is to disturb the problem matrix so that it will change the pattern of its operation for the better.

Also useful are techniques that change current perceptions, so that no matches are made in the problem matrix. This is very relevant when implanting suggestions, because the client must, therefore, be guided to see any post-hypnotic suggestions that you implant as representing change – otherwise their conscious mind won't take any notice of them. Frame the suggestions as changes and get your client to relive them as such, and the effect of the post-hypnotic suggestions will be profound.

Any of the neuro-logical levels can be the chosen target of suggestions, or, indeed, all of them together, using a mudslinging strategy.

Changing the client's beliefs and identity
The suggestions you make should attempt to change your clients' beliefs and identity. Suggestions without evidence or argument to back them up won't work, so, make suggestions that will make them notice a change in their responses and then link it to a change in their identity by use of a complex equivalence. Such linguistic devices are as follows.

	Linguistic form
A = B	That means
A→B	Because

In this way, you are including in your suggestions the changes in their identity, together with the evidence and argument to back them up.

Identify the kind of modification needed
The first thing that you have to do is identify in what way the client's experience and behaviour needs to be modified. Your suggestions will either aim to cause the unconscious not to focus on background data that amounts to the problem, or to see that background information in a different way, so that it does not amount to the problem.

Using trance phenomena in therapy
The best trance phenomena to choose are those of the same type as the client's unconscious mind produces to create the problem.

Age progression
Age progression trance phenomena occur when, in response to problematic childhood conditions, the child age-progresses to a time when they won't have the problem. It enables them to cope.

Repeated use of the age progression trance phenomena makes it become automatic. The *Walter Mitty character* is an extreme case. This is a personality disorder where the individual's behaviour has moved from being context dependent, which is normal, to context independent, which is not, Such individuals are often referred to as dreamers.

The unconscious can't distinguish between the imagined events and real events, because the brain uses the same systems to process them.

Less extreme cases

In less extreme cases the problem arises because of the fact that the unconscious also projects the problem that the child found intolerable into the future, to protect the client against the same kind of events then, by causing the individual to steer clear of such events as cause the current problem.

When any similar event draws near, anxiety is generated to keep the client away from it. The trouble is the generalisation can be far reaching.

This effect is a trance state, because it traps the individual into an inappropriate mode of thinking that belonged in childhood and to a quite different set of circumstance, rather than adulthood and the current circumstances. It is a limiting condition that has happened to the client and they are likely to be aware that it is unwarrantedly affecting them, but feel powerless to avoid or resist the effect. It also involves post hypnotic suggestion, in this case the event that started the problem off.

Using age progression in suggestion

This kind of suggestion is to get the client to imagine a positive future as a consequence of the change they are now making to their thinking. The suggestions aim to bring to the foreground any evidence of change, to convince the client that the problem is moving away.

Regression

This trance phenomenon tends to be the most commonly experienced and is commonly part of a client's problem. It is a core ingredient of panic attacks or any response that resorts to primitive, irrational, or otherwise immature thinking and behaviour.

These are clearly trance states, as they feature all the principle trance characteristics. They are experienced as happening to the individual. They restrict the individual to tunnel vision, as the sufferer can't see outside of their panic and irrational thinking and they involve trance phenomena, notably regression to childhood modes of processing and primary emotions.

Using age regression as a suggestion

Cognitive therapists use this to regress clients to when the problem began in order to help guide them to change their perception of it. Also, age regression can be used to help a client remember past, positive experiences and to get their unconscious to use these as references to future experiences. This improves the client's outlook.

Dissociation
Sometimes a client's problem is rooted in a coping strategy they used as a child to deal with abuse. One such strategy is dissociation. They will have dissociated from a sensation, or emotional feeling, or dissociated from external stimuli

Emotional dissociation
How we deal with emotional states is laid down in childhood, when our parents or other authority figures, create particular experiences in us to go with them. A parent saying, "Big boys don't cry", for example, will lead a child to fear loss of love, if they do and loss of love is arguably the greatest fear of all. The connection between the two things becomes established and thereafter, since that emotional state brings on the fear of loss of love, the individual avoids that emotional state and grows into an emotionally repressed adult.

When anger in childhood is met with a parental response of loss of love, the child may, thenceforth, refuse to accept anger and grow into adulthood as a very passive person, who accepts all manner of abuse from others, without getting wound up about it. The typical image of a butler may spring to mind.

Clinical depression
A neurotic condition that dissociation can result in is clinical depression. This is a response to emotional pain by dissociating from the emotions. The individual becomes numb inside.

Clinical depression brings with it other associated problems, such as loss of appetite, loss of libido, loss of enthusiasm, low self-esteem, underachievement, agoraphobia, lowered immune system effectiveness and other troublesome conditions.

Clinical depression is very clearly a trance state, as it has all the trance ingredients. It is experienced as something that happens to the sufferer. The lines in Keats[33] poem, *Ode to Melancholy* attest to this characteristic being present:

> *"And when the melancholy cloud should fall*
> *sudden from heaven like an April shower"*

Clinical depression restricts the sufferer to tunnel vision and it features the spontaneous emergence of trance phenomena, the obvious one of which is sensory dissociation.

---

[33] Keats (1977)

It is a trance state that you can help your client escape from , but you need to be careful. Consider the consequences. Are they ready to emerge from their psychic sticking plaster – as that's what it is. Have they had a chance to heal inside yet?

Dissociation from external stimuli
When external conditions become intolerable a child may learn to dissociate from the external world. This can manifest itself in excessive internal dialogues, or the creation of an alternative reality. Over time, such a child is likely to grow into a very introverted adult, who feels he, or she is a passive observer of life, rather than a participant.

Psychosomatic illnesses
When, as a result of stress, an individual develops a psychosomatic illness, they have dissociated from reality and this is clearly a trance state, since it contains all the principle trance ingredients. It is experienced as something that has happed to the individual. It restricts their outlook to tunnel vision, as all they can think of is their imaginary illnesses, and it involves the emergence of trance phenomena, notably hallucination (the pain, or illness that isn't really there).

Confusion
A client may present with what appears to be just mental confusion. This, again, is a dissociative condition. The confusion allows the client to disengage from both the emotions and the environmental circumstances with which they cannot, at present, cope, in order to give them time to prepare themselves to handle them.

Using dissociation in therapy
The therapist can use dissociation to keep the client away from their feelings, so that they think, rather than just respond. You need to be alert to any indication that dissociation is part of the problem and to identify what type, or types of dissociation it is.

Use posthypnotic suggestion to direct the client's attention to points in their experience that their neurosis would normally get their mind to delete, distort or generalise, so that you can get them to change that bit of the perception. Use also post-hypnotic suggestion to get the client's mind to notice change in perception and response, so that they positively evaluate the new response.

Post hypnotic suggestion

These are messages we receive in childhood that we continue to unquestionably accept as truth in adulthood. They start as parent → child and become self →self. They become part of the life script that is activated in adulthood. Since these messages are received by our unconscious as post-hypnotic suggestions, the life script is a trance state. Such individuals are living a trance. The therapist's job is to wake them up and show them that this has been the cause of their problem.

If a child is told over and over again (the post hypnotic suggestion), that they are unintelligent they are likely to come to believe it.
Consequently, they will not try to succeed, because they believe they do not have the capability to do so.. This will limit their performance in all walks of life, cause them to underachieve, suffer low self-esteem and other negative effects.

This is clearly a trance state, because it contains all the principal ingredients. It is something that has happened to them. They have tunnel vision, because they cannot see outside of their erroneous self-conception and it features the emergence of trance phenomena, notably post hypnotic suggestion.

Post hypnotic suggestion is also the technique to use to correct this maladaptation. The suggestions should always include an assumption that your client will notice a positive change at some future time

Amnesia as trance phenomena

Amnesia is a defence mechanism that the unconscious mind sometimes employs to protect a child from an experience they cannot process successfully. Psychoanalysts believe amnesia in one form or another is what lies at the root of many neurotic illnesses. When an event is too painful to bear in the consciousness the unconscious may respond by burying the experience in the unconscious and keeping it buried by deterring the individual from any behaviour that might lead to the buried material being uncovered. Amnesia is a severe and all-encompassing form of repression, where the individual can remember nothing at all from before the time when the traumatic experience was buried in the unconscious.

Oedipus and Electra Complexes

The Oedipus complex and the similar Electra complex are typical examples of repression, but psychoanalysts would argue that this repression is a healthy and natural one. In the former, the infant male child's competition with his father, for his mother's love, makes him fear his father will castrate him if he continues to orient himself towards his mother.

In response, he turns away from his mother and identifies with his father. When this stage is completed, the fear of castration is repressed so that the child is never again consciously aware of it. A corresponding process is believed, by psychoanalysts, to take place in the early developmental stage of females.

However, psychoanalysts argue that other traumatic experiences tend to be dealt with in childhood by repression too and in these cases, the repressed memories subsequently cause problems. The memories do not stay passively repressed, their effect bubbles to the surface in the form of anxiety and psychosomatic illnesses, such as asthma, psoriasis, stomach ulcers, and many other forms.

Repression-based maladies are trance states
Such repressions are maladaptations; they do not represent the best way to have handled the traumatic experiences. The symptoms that result from them are trances since they feature all the principal trance phenomena. They are experienced as something that happens to the client. They involve tunnel vision, since the clients are unable to remove themselves from the symptom and they are the product of post hypnotic suggestion. These last two features are definitely the case with psychosomatic illnesses, since these kinds of symptoms tend to disappear as a result of taking placebos – tablets that the client believes are medicants, but which are really nothing more than things like sugar.

Treatment
The therapist can approach the treatment of this kind of malady by Inducing repression. Deliberately inducing repression can often cause a client's mind to go blank. Direct them to focus on the sub-modalities of the blankness, one by one – this often releases the trance and releases the repressed memory, effectively de-hypnotising the client.

Negative hallucination
A negative hallucination is where an aspect of perception is deleted, e.g.

- Conjuring
- Lost keys
- Missed words in a conversation

These are harmless examples, however. Sometimes such a negative hallucination is created by the unconscious to prevent the consciousness from perceiving something that it concludes it would be better off not being aware of. There is none so blind as those who don't want to see, the old saying goes. A benign example of this is not noticing faults in people we love. In fact, when a lover feels their partner has changed it's often just that the clouds of trance have been removed.

The psychoanalytical process known as denial is an example of this, too. Here an individual unconsciously refuses to face up to a truth when the truth is too painful to face.

Because of the tunnel vision nature of trance, negative hallucination is inevitable, because the very fact that the sufferer cannot see outside of the tunnel is a negative hallucination itself.

Disorders that have negative hallucination at their root include things like anorexia nervosa, bulimia, alcoholism, gambling addiction and anger management. Each of these features a tendency, on the part of the sufferer, to deny there is a problem. This is a negative hallucination and the principal obstacle to a cure. Unfortunately, this will also prevent a sufferer seeking help for the same reason and so these are cases that you will not find come your way often.

Another kind of disorder that involves negative hallucination is conversion disorder. This used to be called hysteria, but it has been relabelled. Here the sufferer perceives that they have lost a sensory modality, or a body part. Again, this kind of malady is not very likely to be presented, as another characteristic of this condition is that the sufferer is often unconcerned at the loss they perceive.

Using negative hallucination to treat these conditions.
Instruct your client, under hypnosis, to not notice something different to what they are not noticing now, i.e. the perceptual patch that is obscuring the problem. Direct their attention away from the negative hallucination that the problem that exists is not really there. They will then start to develop amnesia of it and leave the problem to some degree revealed. This should happen, because they are not focussing on it, so it is not generating so much anxiety and there is less unconscious pressure to powerfully deny it.

Use time distortion to create a negative hallucination. Say, for example,

It is not until later that you become aware that you didn't even notice (the thing that was causing the problem).

Positive hallucination
Positive hallucination doesn't infer that this is a positive condition to have. It is referred to as positive only to distinguish it from negative hallucination. The former refers to perceiving something that *is not* really there, while the latter refers to not seeing something that *is*

actually there.   Positive hallucination starts in childhood. Examples are:

- fear of monsters in the dark
- Imaginary friends

All anxiety sufferers are positive hallucinators, because they are responding to something not present, or not known. They are placing something in their future, which may not even be there. Panic attacks are a version of this. These attacks typically last just a couple of minutes, but the extreme fight or flight response activation that takes place leaves the sufferer emotionally and physically exhausted. If these occur often, they may lead to phobophobia - fear of fear, itself.

OCD is another anxiety disorder that involves positive hallucination. The hallucination here is that something terrible will happen if the suffer does not carry out particular rituals.

Phobias feature positive hallucination too. Here the hallucination is that the threat from the phobia object is greater than it actually is. The therapist needs to get the client to create a better hallucination, to cause a distortion of the incoming sensory data, so that they perceive and interpret it positively.

Time distortion
It has been argued that time distortion is a trance state learned in childhood to make bad times pass quickly and vice versa[34]. It could also be a function of the fight or flight response mechanism that dangerous events naturally seem to pass in slow motion. That way we can give more attention to detail, so that we are more likely to survive them.   In good times, endorphins may cause perception to do the reverse. These are ways that this process is adaptive. Time distortion can be utilised by the unconscious in a maladaptive way, though. The unsuccessful periods of the day might be stretched and the successful ones contracted, maybe even so much that they are forgotten, so as to maintain a low level of self-esteem, or lack of confidence.

This is an example of the unconscious getting it wrong. Because an individual feels low self-esteem, or lack of confidence much of the time the unconscious concludes that that is the state with which they know best how to cope. It, therefore, works to ensure that the individual receives perceptions that will reinforce that negative state.

Feelings of low self-esteem and lack of confidence are quite clearly trance states, because they feature the principal trance characteristics.

---

[34] Wolinski (2007)

The individual who suffers from low self-esteem (the feeling that they are not living up to their potential) does not intentionally develop it. The same goes for lack of confidence. These feelings just happen to them, as a result of external influences. The condition locks them in tunnel vision. They are unable to see that this is not the only way to perceive themselves and that the condition has been caused by the continual put-downs of significant others, in the past, which have acted as post-hypnotic suggestions.

The therapist's task is to lead them out of this trance and give them the strength and means of staying outside of it. Once again, the best tool to use is the one that put them in the low self-esteem, or low self-confidence, negative trance in the first place. That instrument is time distortion, the stretched perceptions of their periods of failure and the shrunken perceptions of their periods of success.

Utilising time distortion in therapy
Using time distortion in therapy to overcome this is a pretty straightforward and useful process. You can suggest negative experiences are shorter and positive ones longer, or more frequent. It will suggest to your client that the problem is changeable. You can then negotiate with them to what degree it is changeable

Sensory distortion
Sensory distortion is another trance phenomenon that facilitates certain neurotic symptoms. Examples are:

- Panic attacks
- Phantom limb pain
- Phantom toothache
- Tinnitus
- Anorexia nervosa
- Bulimia

Panic attack is a symptom wherein the heart is perceived to be racing, so much that the individual fears they could even die. Phantom limb and phantom toothache are self-explanatory. Tinnitus is the continued false perception of loud noise in the ears. Anorexia nervosa and bulimia are complicated and multi-causal conditions, the main characteristic of which is a distorted perception of body image. The latter two conditions also have the following features:

- Distortion of satiety feelings, (unwarranted bloatedness or ravenous hunger)
-

- Gustatory distortion (perceiving food as tasting horrible or delightful)

All these conditions are trance states because they all feature the three principal trance characteristics. The individuals do not choose to be in them they just suddenly find the unwelcome symptoms happening to them. They are locked into the symptom by tunnel vision, the result of circular thinking. Thirdly, they are all the result of experiences in the past that have acted as post hypnotic suggestions. The therapist's job is to lead them out of the trance and give them the tools to help them stay out.

Therapeutic use of sensory distortion.
It's easy to fool the senses. You can use sensory distortion techniques to make an imagined cigarette, or piece of chocolate taste bad, or a feeling of nervousness to be perceived as a feeling of anticipation. It's because all sensory data depends on perceptual interpretation, so it's all amenable to distortion.

11

Framing Your Suggestions

So you now know what suggestions to make – the next section informs you how to frame them. The first choice to make is between direct and indirect methods.

Some people are more suggestible than others – those used to obeying orders, such as military personnel, are particularly suited to a direct approach. The scope of this approach is by no means limited to them, though. Particularly stubborn people will respond well to the indirect approach. Again, though, this approach is by no means limited to that group.

Direct suggestion
Direct suggestion is where the therapist tells the client what they will do, feel and experience.

Indirect suggestion.
The formulation of indirect suggestions involves what can best be described as artful vagueness.

The assumption from the outset, in the latter case, is that the clients have the resources to heal themselves and, with guidance, can find and access them. Formulate a clear idea of what you want your client to achieve and then help them do so, in a very flexible way. Give them minimal guidance and let them fill in the blanks, so that they are largely finding their own way there.

By use of vague and ambiguous language, you can induce clients to look for the meanings of your words within their own deep structure and discover, there, the mental resources they need to relieve their problem. Therapists call this the transcendental search or TDS.

The TDS is, itself, trance inducing, because of its inward focus, and it can send the client into a trance state even before formal induction.

The Milton Model
The Milton model is a series of language patterns that are available to a hypnotherapist, by the use of which they will be able to pace and lead their client's behaviour, distract their consciousness and so gain

direct access to and communication with their unconscious. Those patterns include:

- Presuppositions (Implying that you know what they are thinking)
- Lost performatives
- Cause and effect
- Complex equivalence
- Awareness
- Universal quantifiers
- Modal operators that imply possibility
- Nominalisations
- Unspecified verbs
- Tag questions
- Lack of referential index
- Binds
- Double binds
- Protracted series of quotations
- Ambiguous forms
- Uncertainty of how much of a sentence descriptions are meant to apply to
- Utilisation of context
- Embedded commands
- Pacing words to client's manifest behaviour

Presuppositions

Presuppositions are linguistic equivalents of assumptions. Using presuppositions, you can make the unconscious accept something unwittingly, thereby avoiding resistance.

Presuppositions of possibility

Words such as: *may, might* and *could* presuppose possibility.

Presuppositions of time

Using presuppositions of time is very powerful. These forms include words such as continue, e.g. *As you continue to develop confidence in yourself.*

They are powerful because they shift attention away from whether the client will, or will not do so. It is that doubt that creates anxiety and this perpetuates and, perhaps, increases their self-doubt. By shifting away from this question that acts as a barrier to acceptance a post-hypnotic suggestion of confidence is allowed to be accepted.

Words that can be used for inserting time presuppositions include: *already, anymore, begin, end, start, stop, continue, still and yet.*

Presuppositions of successful change
Use of an appropriate adverb to draw focal attention away from an important term in a hypnotic suggestion will also help to avoid resistance. Here are some examples:

...how surprisingly calm you are in its presence
...how calmly and confidently you resist the unreasonable demands of your boss
 ...how unusually calm and confident you feel in the presence of the group
...how easily you resist the temptation to smoke.

Ordinal presuppositions
Ordinal presuppositions are presuppositions of repetition of something. They can be expressed in words such as: *first, second, thirdly, fourthly, next*, etc. They presuppose that whatever state is being suggested to exist it is not the first time that it has existed.

Here are some examples

You may not fully notice how much your confidence has been growing until the third, or even the fourth time you present your lecture.

It may not be until after the second, or third meal that you first become aware that you have had no desire to smoke after any of the previous meals.

Presuppositions of existence
Presuppositions of existence are induced by language that takes them for granted without actually saying them, for example, you might say to your client:

You might look at those going outside, in the cold, for a cigarette with pity, because you feel no such craving yourself.

Implying that you know, what they are thinking and feeling
Vague mind reading implications by the therapist add to the client's sense of confusion about the data they are receiving from the outside world. This reinforces their tendency to turn their attention inwards. An example of such forms is:

And you are wondering where your mind will take you next.

Lost performatives

Lost performatives are value judgements without stating whose values, as if they are universally held and self-evident. Here are some examples:

- *It is good to let your mind wander.*
- *It's good to feel highly about yourself.*
- *It's good to have ambition.*

Cause and effect

Cause and effect suggestions are important, because suggestions will be accepted more readily and strongly if there is evidence to back them up. You can present this evidence by use of cause and effect suggestions. The suggestions will include terms such as: *Because you..., If...then* and *As you...then you*

Bandler suggested there are three discernible levels on which cause and effect suggestions can be made:

Level I - A weak causal linkage is made by use of the conjunction *and*. An example is:
Your breathing is slowing and you are beginning to relax.

Level II - The conjunction here implies a time sequence between one thing and the other. Examples are:
When your mind is ready to do some important inner work you can step off the bottom step of the staircase and enter into your own wonderful place of relaxation.
...and while you continue to focus on my words, so your eyelids are becoming ever more tired.

Level III - Here the suggestion actually states the causal linkage, for example:
Each out-breath makes your eyelids become more tightly locked together.

Complex equivalence

A complex equivalence is a suggestion that two things are equated, such as:
You may notice how relaxed you become and that means that your unconscious mind has become ready to make important changes.

Complex equivalence suggestions employ terms such as: *This means..., That means...,* and *Which means... .*

Awareness
Use awareness to guide your client's unconscious to become aware of some sensory data or other, for example, *You may be aware of a feeling of relaxation.*

Universal quantifiers
Universal quantifiers are words such as: *all, any, always, each, every, nowhere, never,* etc. These are used to generalise your client's experience.

Modal operators that imply possibility
Modal operators implying possibility include words such as: *Can, could, may, might, should and will.* The value of modal operators is that they avoid resistance, because they do not suggest that the client is feeling or thinking anything, but merely that it is possible for them to do so. Here are some examples of their use:

And you might notice, your eyelids becoming heavy and tired.You may feel a twitch in your elbow, or the slightest movement of your thumb."

You might feel the slightest tremor in a finger, as your hand begins gently to raise itself off your lap.

Nominalisations
Nominalisations are abstract nouns, such as: *knowledge, understanding, learning,* etc. The therapist can use these to guide a client to explore their inner self and their problem.

Unspecified verbs
Unspecified verbs, such as: *change, grasp, feel, learn, know, think, understand and wonder,* when left without stated objects lead the client to provide the latter. This draws them into the trance, bypassing resistance.

TAG questions
Tag questions are questions that are tagged on to the end of a suggestion. They serve to bypass resistance. Here is an example:

You are aware of the damage smoking does to your health, aren't you?

Lack of referential index
Suggestions deliberately lacking a referential index are similar to those of unspecified verbs, except that here it is a whole phrase or sentence that is missing, leaving the client to supply this from their

own mind. Again, forms such as this serve to bypass resistance. An example is:

It is a change you are making in your own psyche.

Pacing words to clients manifest behaviour

It is useful to link your words to the behaviour of your client, because they will be less incongruent and, therefore, less likely to meet resistance. The congruence will lull the client into a relaxed state. An example is:

And as you move to arrange your body into a more comfortable position, so your unconscious is moving its contents into a more comfortable and appropriate configuration, so that the inappropriate structures of thinking no longer exist in it.

Binds

There are single and double binds (sometimes called *exclusive or* presuppositions). Single binds are alternatives presented to the client, both of which will lead their mind in the direction you want it to go. When offered a pair of alternative courses of action most people will not consider that they can accept neither option and will instead, choose one of them. This is a very powerful way to lead a person' thinking. It is a favourite of sales representatives; they call it the binary choice close. When they ask,

Which one are you going to have, this one or that one?,

many buyers will choose one or the other, because they have not been given the choice of neither of them. What is actually being offered is only the illusion of choice, for whichever they choose the result will be the same.

In therapy this can be used to convince the client that some degree of change has already taken place by, for example, suggesting that they may notice a large change, or a small change in their level of confidence. It prevents them considering a third option, i.e. that no change has occurred. It shifts their focus onto just how much change has occurred, away from whether or not, any change has occurred at all.

Double bind

Double binds are suggestions that particular conditions will evoke an automatic response. There are several classes of these:

- Time – behaviour.
- Dissociation
- Double dissociation

Time – behaviour double binds
Time – behaviour double binds are suggestions implanted that a future point in time will trigger a particular autonomic response. A classic example of this is its usage by Milton Erickson as follows:

I know your father and mother have been asking you, Jimmy, to quit biting your nails. They don't seem to know that you are just a six-year-old boy and they don't seem to know that you will naturally quit biting your nails, just before you're seven years old..."

Other examples are:

And it might not be until after you have not smoked for 3 days that you become fully aware that you have not missed cigarettes at all.

It may not be until just before the interview that you become fully aware of just how confident you are of making a good impression on the panel.

Dissociation double bind
The dissociation double blind works by splitting the functions of the conscious and the unconscious minds. Here are a couple of example:

And it really doesn't matter whether you're consciously hearing, what I'm saying, as your unconscious mind will be taking it in and responding to it.

And it really doesn't matter whether or not you're aware of what your unconscious mind is learning from my words.

Using protracted series of quotations
By couching the suggestion within a quotation or statement made by someone else, you can avoid the critical judgement with which the suggestion would otherwise be received and modified. It can, thus, be implanted unaffected by resistance in the same way as powerful enduring suggestions are received from parents before the age when critical thinking develops. The quotation might be from an authority figure or a client or, better still, a statement or quotation made by someone about something they had heard from someone else, as the longer the chain of abstraction the better. The avoidance of critical judgement happens because the chain of origination of the idea causes them to lose interest in evaluating it and it is thus absorbed unmodified.

Anthropomorphism
Anthropomorphism is attributing animal qualities and abilities to non-living things, for example:

And as that chair feels the weight of your body relaxing gently into its soft cushions...

These kinds of constructions build confusion and, thus, deepen the trance.

Using ambiguous forms

Clever use of ambiguous forms can enable you to make your client think that a suggestion you have made, or advice you have given actually came from they themselves, thereby removing or reducing resistance. There are various kinds of ambiguous forms, you can choose.

Ambiguity of syntax

Ambiguity of syntax refers to where a word or phrase, placed at a particular place in a sentence, gives rise to alternative meanings. Here is an example:

...and you may now be surprised at how confident you are aware at last of your real ability.

Ambiguity of parts of speech

Ambiguity can be introduced by phrasing suggestions so that a word can be taken as either a verb or an adjective. Here are some examples:

Following events will be equally successful

Reassuring people can help

Loving friends will help you through

Ambiguity of sound

Words that have similar phonological sounds but different meanings can be used in sentences that provide a different message for each version of the phoneme. An example is:

... and as you continue to relax your mind might just wonder (wander) where it is even more   relaxing still.

Uncertain objects of epithets

You can create uncertainty of how much of a sentence describing words are meant to apply to and use this to deepen the trance. An example of this kind of ambiguity is:

... and those heavy eyelids and arms sink down further.

Utilisation of context

It is important to utilise the environmental perceptions that will be reaching your client during the induction and trance. This will reduce incongruity and prevent weakening of the trance as a result of the client's attention turning towards the outer world. It will also increase the congruity of your suggestions. Here is an example of such utilisation:

And as you hear the wind blowing outside, so you can feel your hang-ups drifting away with the wind.

Inserting embedded commands

Inserting embedded commands is a powerful tactic in hypnotherapy and used almost universally by competent hypnotists. It involves changing the tone of voice when particular words are spoken, words which would otherwise not appear to be authoritative commands. Here is an example:

*... and now that you have decided to **stop smoking**, you can begin to enjoy better health.*

Using reverse psychology in posthypnotic suggestion

If you tell someone not to do something they will be more likely to actually do it. If what you tell them to do is not to think of something in particular at a particular time, or on a particular cue, then they will almost certainly do the opposite. They will think of the thing you told them not to think of. This is because we can't remember not to think of something without remembering what it is we are not supposed to think of. Consequently, you can plant very powerful suggestions in this way. Here is an example:

When you finish your breakfast tomorrow morning, and every morning after that, you are not to remember the images of diseased lungs and the long list of dangerous chemicals in cigarettes.

If you have used aversion therapy, you can add the command that they are not to remember the smell of vomit, or whatever other aversive stimulus you have used.

Involving a positive state in a posthypnotic suggestion

By implanting a suggestion that will induce a positive emotion on the happening of some event, the appearance of that emotion should prevent the emergence of a negative emotional state. This is because two opposing states cannot coexist at the same time. Here's an example:

... and you may feel surprised at the acute sense of concentration you feel as you walk onto the stage, which makes you realise that you feel totally confident to present your lecture.

12

Subconscious Relearning

This stage of the therapy process involves asking the client to describe his or her new understanding of what was previously a problem. The goal is to ensure that the client achieves a more mature and appropriate understanding of the situation, the problem, its cause and the solution.

If this is, itself, done under trance conditions the verbalisation and the therapist's paraphrasing and relaying back to the client will have maximum effect. The therapist should employ imagery, metaphor and symbol in their paraphrasings, because this is the language that the unconscious mind understands.

The trance state makes the client more suggestible and if the material is coming from the client him, or herself, albeit paraphrased by the therapist, it will not meet with resistance. If there is any negative response it will suggest that more therapy is required.

Relearning can be facilitated at intermediate stages in the therapy, or all at once at the end.

Here are some examples of the words a therapist might use:

... and I want you to tell me how you now feel about the issue, with the new insights and awareness that you now have.

How will these new understandings affect the way that you deal with the issue and how will it affect your life in general, both now and in the future?

You can, alternatively, lead your client, under trance conditions, to their peaceful place and ask their unconscious mind to reveal the new awareness to the consciousness by ideomotor responses (the 'yes' finger, for example)

When you are paraphrasing, reinforcing and relaying back your client's verbalisations you can adjust your style to that to which your client responds best. If they respond best to direct suggestion then relate what you say back to them in the second person form. If they respond best to indirect suggestion, then couch your paraphrasing in indirect language.

Inappropriate new understandings
If any of the new understandings verbalised by the client seem inappropriate suggest that it could be talked over at a conscious level first.

13

Ego Strengthening

Ego strengthening reinforces progress in therapy. It is, therefore, recommended that this procedure is carried out after every treatment, prior to bringing the client out of the trance. It enhances the positive feelings that the client associates with trance states. It also strengthens the rapport between the therapist and client, which is a crucial condition of successful hypnotherapy.

The usual method is for the therapist to make a serious of authoritative suggestions. These are very general and all-encompassing and do not require any tailoring to suit the client's hypnotic suggestibility level. The most important factor in their success is likely to be the rapport and confidence in the therapist already built up and the quality of the therapy so far received.

A note of caution

Ego strengthening should not be relied upon as the sole therapeutic procedure in the treatment of mood disorders. It can be useful on its own for treating stress and anxiety[35], but overdependence on it in the treatment of mood disorders can prove dangerous. Heap[36] reports a case where ego-strengthening procedure by a lay therapist resulted in a suicide attempt by the client.

Here is a typical ego strengthening script that I, and many others, were taught many years ago during our own training and one which is used by many, many practitioners to this day.

You have now become so deeply relaxed... so deeply comfortable... that your mind has become so sensitive... so receptive to what I say... that everything we discuss... will sink so deeply into the unconscious part of your mind... and will cause such a deep and lasting impression there... that it will become a part of your new everyday reality.

Consequently, these new learnings that your unconscious mind makes... will begin to exercise a greater and greater influence over

---

[35] Stanton (1990)
[36] ___ (1984)

the way you think... over the way you feel... over the way you behave... and will fit your life in a manner that will truly meet your needs.

So that as a result of your inner experience in the trance today... as each day goes by you are going to feel physically stronger and fitter in every way... you will feel more alert... more focused... more optimistic... than you have felt in a long... long while.

Every day, you will become more calm and clear in your mind... and relaxed in your body... You will become so much more deeply interested in whatever you are doing... in whatever is going on around you... that your mind's attention... for long periods will be completely distracted away from yourself...

And this will mean that even if the occasional worry or concern comes your way... which will be much less... you can just allow it to pass... so that quickly and easily it will be followed by other thoughts and feelings... that seem so much more helpful... so that... instantly your attention will be directed somewhere else... somewhere more appropriate... because you allow that process to happen...

And as a result of your inner rest and rejuvenation period in the trance... every day... your nerves will become stronger and steadier... which will mean your mind becomes calmer and clearer... more composed... more tranquil... and much more able to cope... with whatever you encounter in your daily life.

You will be able to think more clearly... you will be able to concentrate more easily... you will be able to give your whole undivided attention to whatever you are doing... to the complete exclusion of any unwanted distractions... consequently... your memory will improve... and so will your ability to concentrate for much longer periods...

And you will be able to see situations and events in your life in their true perspective... and in a way in which you can cope and deal with effectively.
Every day you we will become emotionally much calmer... and much more settled...

And as you become... and as you remain... more relaxed... and calm as each day goes by... so... you will develop much more confidence in yourself... more self-confidence in your ability to do... not only what you have to do each day... but more confidence in your inner ability to do whatever you wish to do... to challenge... and go beyond limiting beliefs of the past... to create new experiences... and naturally you will expand your world... and develop much more belief in yourself...

And because of these natural changes... every day... you will feel more and more independent...more able to stand up for yourself... to stand on your own feet... to rely on your own opinions and *judgements... and then back yourself up... in whatever decisions you choose to make...*

Every day... you will feel a greater feeling of personal well-being... both physical as well as mental well-being... a greater feeling of personal safety and security... than you have felt in a long... long time.

14

Bringing the Client Out of the Trance

The final part of the therapy session is bringing the client out of the trance. This is usually referred to as *waking*, although it is a misnomer, because waking implies that the client has been asleep. If they had been the therapy would not be very successful. The hypnotic state is a conscious, but highly relaxed and receptive state, but not a snooze.

The task for the therapist, in this procedure, is to reverse all the effects of the hypnosis except for the therapy effects, i.e.. the discoveries, the suggestions, the relearnings and the ego strengthening. Be sure to reverse any non-therapeutic suggestions you used, for example, suggestions that you may have used to deepen the trance, such as:

As the clock chimes you go deeply into the trance
or
When I snap my fingers like this you will go immediately back into the trance.

Even if there seemed to be no response to such suggestions during the induction or therapy session, reverse the suggestions anyway, as the unconscious is capable of delayed response.

If parts therapy has been used all the parts of the body and mind now need to be reintegrated. The body and mind must be returned to experiencing normal sensations. If regression has been involved then it is important to return the client firmly to the present.

If you have used the out of body induction and deepening technique, you must reintegrate your client before bringing them out of the trance. To do so, proceed as follows:

And when every part of you is back inside... every part of you back here in the present with me... and you have completed as much inner work as is appropriate for you at this time... you can gently allow your eyes to open... stretch and feel refreshed.

A final ego boost can be incorporated into the communication with the entranced client if you wish.

It can be useful to use a different tone and/or tempo of voice to wake a client from the trance. This is to signal, clearly, to the client's mind that there is a difference between the trance world and waking life.

Alternatively, you may progressively change the tone and tempo to signal that the client is going through the transition from one to the other.

Here is a typical waking script that I learned many years ago, when I was training and I still use this, or something similar, today.

And now...I'm going to wake you.... In a few seconds time... you'll hear me count... from one to ten.... You will slowly come awake... with each number ... and at the count of eight... you will open your eyes... and by the count of ten,... you will be fully wide-awake.... You will wake up feeling fine ... with a feeling of well-being...all over ... feeling of well-being.... Every part of you will be back here with me in the present... and you will be fully wide-awake at the count of ten.... You will feel fine... refreshed ... feeling better... feeling more confident... and more optimistic too... than you have felt in a long, long while.... So... as I count from one to ten... so you come more and more awake with each number... and at the count of eight... you will open your eyes ... and at the count of ten... you will be fully wide awake....

... So ... ready... one ... two...three... WAKING UP-... four... five ... six... WAKING UP... seven.... eight ...OPEN YOUR EYES... nine...ten... WIDE-AWAKE... WIDE-AWAKE... WIDE-AWAKE... Stretch and feel refreshed.

15

Managing Your Practice

Managing a hypnotherapy practice is basically like managing any other business. The principles are the same. You seek to make a living by providing an expert service and to reap rewards from it in order to fulfil your lifestyle aspirations. Therefore, you have to plan, price, promote and distribute your want- satisfying services to present and potential customers[37]. Let's deal with each of these in turn.

Planning your services

What service are you going to offer? Is it gastric band therapy, a quick fix for phobias, economy quit smoking sessions, some other specialism, or are you going to operate a general surgery as a therapist. You have to make up your mind on this, as you can't be all things to all segments of the market. It just doesn't work. You will just end up diluting the value of advertising and promotion.

At whom are you aiming your services?

You need to decide to which segment of the market you are pitching. Is it the rich and famous, or the man on the Clapham omnibus? Again, you have to make a decision here, as you can't share an advertising budget between segments of the market, without diluting it. Furthermore, the image you portray trying to attract one group may deter another group.

Pricing your service

You also need to decide how much you are going to charge. Pricing is not just a simple matter of *the cheaper you set your prices the more customers you'll get.*

There is a price-plausibility curve that relates the plausibility of your message to the price you are charging and it's not straightforward. If you envisage a continuum between the minimum and maximum prices that hypnotherapists charge, at the top end of the scale potential clients will want the maximum amount of *information* before they will buy it,

---

[37] Stanton (1981)

but at the bottom end they will need the maximum amount of *explanation* as to why it is so cheap.

It's best to set you price somewhere in the middle of the curve, unless you can supply a plausible explanation for offering services on the cheap, or there is already ample information out there that warrants a disproportionately high fee level.

Advertising
A good advertising strategy has two parts

- Media strategy
- Copy strategy

Media Strategy
The media strategy is the choice of media to use. This, again, is not a simple matter. A lot of money is wasted on advertising , even in large organisations, simply because their message does not reach the target group in sufficient quantity, or with a sufficient quality of readership that the cost justifies the expenditure. A lot of advertising decisions are made on a whim, or in response to an advertising sales rep's call.

It's best to research carefully which media is aimed at your target group. Such statistics are available in media guides that are available in libraries and on the internet. Willings Press Guide[38] is an example. This is why it is so important, initially, to establish exactly at whom you are aiming your services, i.e. your target group.

Cost/benefit analysis
The advertising costs vary widely between different media. Therefore, it's not just a case of choosing the one that reaches the highest number of people in the target group, in your area. If the advertising price is high the costs may outweigh the benefits. The yardstick to use is the *lowest cost per 1000 exposures to the target group.*

Readership quality
Nor is it simple even then, because the message might reach your target group, but they might not read it or, if they do, they might just notice the title and skip over it. It is important to assess the likely readership quality. Small ads in newspapers for hypnotherapy sessions will not attract much attention, though press articles with an interesting story to tell will. In the latter case, you can add a bi-line at the end, advertising your practice.

---

[38] Warwick (2012)

Leaflets are another option, but although the unit cost is relatively small and exposure to the target group relatively high, if you distribute them appropriately, the response rate is not that good. You will be lucky to get one enquiry per thousand leaflets, so you have to balance the net income value of one new client against the cost of printing and delivering 1000 leaflets.

One medium where you are likely to attract the focussed attention of the man on the Clapham omnibus is on the Clapham omnibus – on the interior wall, where advertising posters are displayed. Another place is on the walls of the bus shelter where he waits for the bus.

The reason this medium is so powerful is not only that it reaches your target group, if that is the target group you have chosen, but, more importantly, the quality of readership will be high. This is because people who are travelling on buses , trains and planes are bored and looking for something to occupy their mind. They will read absolutely anything, word for word.

Of course, the owners of the transport and all that goes with it – bus shelters, railway platforms and airport lounges - know how valuable it is and charge accordingly, so while the exposure and readership quality is high, so is the price. You have to consider whether it is worth it and your yardstick is the formula *lowest cost per thousand exposures to the target group*, adjusting for an assessment of readership quality.

Other sites with the same quality
There are, however, other transportation type media that are not expensive and it is here that you can often find the best of both worlds – low price and high readership quality. Transportation advertising is something of a misnomer, because sometimes the media that fall into this category have nothing to do with transport. They come under the heading because they have the same quality as bus shelter and railway platform adverts – their viewers are waiting for something and are bored.

Doctors and dentists surgeries, therefore, come into this category. Anywhere where people have to wait offers such an opportunity of value for money advertising, whether it is by means of posters on the walls , or flyers on the tables. In some cases there will be no charge at all, though you will be expected to obtain permission, unless there is a free notice board policy.

The Internet
Many hypnotherapists now rely, considerably, on the Internet to advertise their services. A basic website can be designed and produced for you for about £500. This will give you a lot of scope to present

every aspect of your business and every competitive advantage you feel you have.

Copy strategy

Having decided where you are going to advertise, you have to work out what you are going to say. Again, this can be split into two main categories.

- Informational advertising
- Persuasive advertising

Informational advertising

If people don't know you are there or what you do then there is no chance that they will use your services. You have to make the basic information available to the target group - your name, where you are, what you are qualified to do and the services you offer.

General directories, such as the phone book and specialist directories, such as lists of hypnotherapists, are places where you can make this information available. A sign outside your consulting rooms, or a well-designed facia will also present some basic information to passers-by. You might also inform local doctors, dentists. sports clubs and so on, so that they might mention your practice to patients. They won't actually recommend you, however, until they know you and know something about how competent you are.

Persuasive advertising

As a hypnotherapist, you are working in the private sector of the health care market, so you've got to be prepared to compete with others. Competition is good; it keeps everyone on their toes and works towards ensuring that clients get the best value for money. If you're good you need to get the message across to potential clients that yours is the practice they should choose.

The tangible and Intangible messages

There are two parts to the message - the tangible and the intangible. The tangible image is the message you are sending to their conscious mind. It's the message that spells out, literally, why they should choose your practice rather than someone else's. It contains what marketing people call your USPs - unique selling points.

- You might specialise in a particular procedure
- You might be particularly highly qualified
- You may have been practising for a long time

- You may have illustrious clients (though never name them)
- Your services may be affordable to the average person
- You may have a surgery that is worth boasting about

The intangible message

The second part of the message is the intangible image. As a hypnotherapist, you know, more than most, that it is the unconscious that is the most powerful driver of human, choice behaviour. You also know that the language of the unconscious is not verbal but, rather, imagery, metaphor and symbol. Therefore, if you want your message to really hit home you might think about how you are going to reinforce what you have said verbally in the language of the unconscious.

Consider which colour, for example, suggests caring and healing - many consider this to be mauves. Consider whether you might employ the archetypal symbols of the healer (one of Jung's archetypes). You might include images of smiling people, expressing liberation from a phobia, or addiction, or even a short comic strip, telling a story of how they have benefitted from your service. Imagery, remember, is a language the unconscious understands.

Point of sale promotion.

Point of sale promotion is not as relevant to this service as it is to many other services in the market place. When you have successfully treated a client's malady it's not really appropriate to expect, or encourage another need for therapy. You would, arguably, be encouraging a dependency.

However, promotional materials, such as pens, calendars and so on can be useful gifts to people who may recommend your services in the future - doctors, dentists, sports coaches and so on. It will help keep your name in their mind.

Business cards

Business cards are a must. Some therapists have the back of the cards printed to act as appointment cards. This is not a bad idea.

In order to get referrals from doctors, you will need to contact them and convince them of the worthwhileness of recommending your services to clients. Initial letters to the surgery, introducing your services, are likely to be binned straight away and you will have to follow them up in other ways to get their attention.

Staff

It is favourable to have another person present in the practice when providing therapy, for all sorts of reasons. Unless your partner is going to act as receptionist, you may consider employing someone. If you do, you'll need to know something about:

- Recruitment
- Health and safety at work
- Personnel management
- PAYE
- Dismissal procedures

The media available for advertising such a job incudes:

- Job centres
- Local newspapers
- Gum tree website
- Employment agencies

You will need to compile:

- Job specification
- Candidate profile
- Application form.

The job specification is a statement of what the candidate will be required to do and it should be comprehensive. The candidate profile is a statement of the abilities, qualities, knowledge and skills the successful candidate will have.

In addition to a completed application form, some employers ask for a CV. This is a statement of the facts the *candidate* wants to tell you, while the completed application form will contain what *you* want them to tell you.

When you interview a candidate it is advisable to ask them for examples of when they have demonstrated the abilities, qualities, knowledge and skills that you expect the successful candidate to have. It's advisable to ask for employers' references if the candidate has had previous jobs and if you offer them the job make it dependent upon the receipt of satisfactory references.

What qualities would you need in a receptionist/assistant?
The qualities that you ought to seek in a candidate would be punctuality, reliably, honesty, discretion, confidentiality, cleanliness and smart appearance. They ought to have good communication skills and adequate office administration skills.

Their usefulness to you will, to some extent, depend on the way they are treated and their working conditions.

Salary level determines the likelihood that an employee will stay, but this alone will not motivate them to work efficient and productively. What determines this is working conditions – how happy the worker is in their work and their workplace.

The decor and ambience of the office and the quality of their desk and chair are all factors of this. The manner in which you treat them is also important. If you are interested in them, in their professional development, they will be interested in you and your business. They will work in your interests if they like you; they may be less likely to do so if they don't.

Health and safety

There are health and safety considerations with which you need to familiarise yourself. The subject in any great depth is beyond the scope of this book.

Other considerations

There should be a complaints procedure, so that the employee knows exactly what they must do if they are not happy with something. This prevents bad feelings festering when a person does not know how to complain when they feel it is justified.

Regular reviews of their progress should be carried out and feedback given. Not only does this ensure the employee is performing as they should, but it communicates to the employee that you are interested in their development.

Accounts

Unless you are well skilled in bookkeeping and accounting, it is advisable to employ an accountant from the word go. You'll need to account for fee income, expenses and asset purchases on a regular basis.

Fee income will be a simple matter of keeping a fee income daybook. If you are not permitting credit accounts, then there is no need for a client ledger. Expenditure will first be recorded in a purchase daybook. Bankings will be recorded in the bank cashbook. If you have some bookkeeping skills, you may wish to do the next stage of the accounts in posting the details from the daybooks to the nominal and bought divisions of the ledger, but, if you haven't the skills, you can employ the services of a freelance bookkeeper to do this. They will charge a monthly fee, typically about £50 per month.

Administration

It's advisable to ask clients for payment before they receive their treatment, as you want the effect of the treatment to continue after they leave the consulting room, uninterrupted by any thoughts in their mind about the expenditure.

Your receptionist should greet clients warmly and professionally and ensure they are seated comfortably while they wait to be shown into your consulting room. If they have to wait more than a few minutes then they might offer them a cup of tea or coffee.

Record keeping in such practices used to be done on cards but, nowadays, a MS Access program will make it easier and take up less space. It goes without saying that records should be kept accurately, but the Data Protection Act restricts the amount of data that can be held on a person. You need to familiarise yourself with this. This act also places strict requirements of confidentiality on all those with access to this data.

Presentation of your business premises

Obviously, the quality of your premises is important. The client will not feel confident if you operate from a shabby, backstreet office. One way of ensuring that your premises make a good impression on your clients is to rent space in a general therapy practice. These practices, however, typically charge 40 to 50% of fees.

What should you have in your consulting room? It is advisable to make your consulting room look the part. Ideally, there should be a desk, but you should avoid sitting behind it when the client is present, unless you are doing purely administrative tasks, like writing out a bill, or a receipt for payment, or making an entry in the appointments book.

There should be comfortable seats in the room. Ideally, there should be a recliner chair, or a couch and at least a couple of other comfortable chairs.

Your qualification certificates should be displayed on the walls, as also should be your certificates of membership of professional bodies, your certificate of professional indemnity insurance and any other certificates required by law to be displayed in business premises.

The consulting room should be warm, but not stifling. Extremes of both cold and heat make people uncomfortable and that will work against the successful therapy.

Before you begin therapy

As much soundproofing as is reasonably achievable should be done. Double-glazing has a very significant effect in reducing noise from the outside.

Relevant information leaflets can be placed around, for example, information about particular conditions with which hypnotherapists deal. These are usually available from associations dedicated to the particular conditions.

Any relevant posters which give information about particular conditions, or about hypnotherapy generally will add to the favourable impression the client receives, as will, of course, any press articles that extol the virtues and achievements of hypnotherapy.

There ought to be a feature upon the wall, which you can use as a focal point in induction, perhaps a spot on the wall or the ceiling, if you intend to use methods that require this,.

Ethical practice.

Guidelines for ethical practice

1. Don't Induce unrealistic expectations
2. Don't attempt to treat people for problems with which you are unfamiliar
3. Don't overstep boundaries of competence
4. Always enquire about psychological and medical history and any current medications
5. Don't treat people who are already under treatment for this or a related condition by another practitioner without the consent of that other practitioner
6. Avoid using inappropriate methods of hypnotherapy
7. Never give guarantees of success. It would be unethical to do so as success cannot be guaranteed in hypnotherapy. If a client does not want to be hypnotised or successfully treated they won't be. They are in control; you assure them of this from the outset, so to claim guaranteed success is simply dishonest and misrepresents the service you can offer.
8. Don't breach confidentiality, if you wish to discuss a client symptoms, treatment or progress with colleagues change the name you use for the patient.
9. Never suggest that the patient should stop medication for any condition
10. Never reproach other medical professionals they are seeing
11. Keep treatment times as short as possible. "Treat and street" is a saying that I think is apt. Clients can develop a dependency on the therapist if the treatment is prolonged beyond the time necessary for cure. You would be acting in contradiction of your professional purpose if you allow this to happen.

12. Training should be on-going. There are new developments taking place, from time to time and a good therapist will wish to keep up to date. In addition, skills get rusty if they are not used and refresher courses can keep them up to cutting-edge proficiency.
13. It is vital to be adequately covered by a professional indemnity insurance policy. It is also advisable to hold a membership of a regulatory body.

Dealing with the initial appointment call

I would recommend that you keep your appointment booking call brief. This is time you are not being paid for, so don't get into a consultation situation on the phone. Spend no more than five minutes at the most on the phone. Also, be efficient, concise and business-like. Take control of the conversation – don't just listen and let the prospective client control it. The only things you need to deal with are:

- What the problem is.
- Tell them whether you can help.
- Tell them what you charge
- Arrange the appointment time
- Take down the client's name and phone number
- Give directions to your practice.
- Ask where they got your details from
- Inform them of the conditions for changing appointments

Let's deal with each of these in a bit more detail.

When the caller tells you what the problem is, if you are not certain whether you can help without further information tell them that they should have a 1 - 1½ hour consultation in the first instance, where you can take a case history and investigate the problem further. You will then be able to tell them whether you will be able to help. Inform them that there are never any guarantees. It is on the second session that you can decide exactly what techniques you will use; you have a range of them at your disposal.

If they ask what hypnotherapy is just explain that it is basically therapy while in a very receptive state of mind, but it will all be fully explained to them at the time.

If they ask you how long it will take to resolve the problem tell them that they can expect some change after the first session but you can't tell them how much. Everyone is different. Explain that the aim is to get them on the road to recovery as soon as possible and then say goodbye. Tell them you don't do long-term therapy.

Avoid negotiation on charges. This is the first stage of allowing yourself to be manipulated and the hypnotherapist must stay in control. This is crucial to the relationship between hypnotherapist and client and the success of the therapy.

Ask them when they want to make an appointment for. Don't make appointments for more than two weeks ahead; they are likely to be missed. If they want to make an appointment more than two weeks ahead ask them to call back nearer the time.

Take down their name, address and phone number. Expect 10% hoax calls. Give precise directions on how to get to the practice, as this will help reduce lateness.

Before commencing therapy

Before you begin therapy, make sure you switch off the phone. It is also a good idea to have a switch to disconnect the doorbell. You might also have a notice displayed on the door saying *Therapy in progress. Please do not disturb between ___and ___ times*. If you have a receptionist, or are renting rooms in a therapy centre disturbances such as this will not, or should not occur.

The first session will usually have the greatest effect. If no improvement is seen after the first session then, unless you have other techniques to try, you should really suggest that, with the procedures you have, they are not ready to make the changes. Suggest referring to another kind of therapist, if appropriate.

Ending the therapy

When you feel you have made the necessary improvement tell the client so and suggest that there is now a window to see how they manage. They can call you in a month, if they are still having problems.

Bibliography

Ader, R. (2007) ed. Psychoneuroimmunology, LONDON: Elsevier.

Bateson, G. (1972) Steps to an ecology of mind, LONDON: Paladin.

Barnard, J. (1977) ed. John Keats: The Complete Poems, LONDON: Penguin.

Bernheim. H. (2010) Suggestive therapeutics; A treatise on the nature and uses of hypnotism, LONDON: London Book Co.

Braid, J. (2012) Neurypnology, or the rationale of nervous sleep, considered in relation with animal magnetism, MASSACHUSETTS: Hard Press Publishing.

Breuer, J. (2000) Studies on hysteria, NEW YORK: Basic Books.

Cannon, W. B. (1929). Bodily changes in pain, hunger, fear, and rage, NEW YORK:Appleton-Century-Crofts.

Coue, E. (2006) Self mastery through conscious autosuggestion, MONTANA: Kessinger

Ellenberger, H. (1970) Discovery of the unconscious: The history and evolution of dynamic psychiatry, NEW YORK: Basic Books. pp. 70-74,

Esdaile, J., Elliotson J. and Macnish, R. (1977) sleep, CONNECTICUT: Praeger.

Faria Abbe (2006) The master of hypnotism who charmed Napoleon, NEW DELHI: Ritana Books.

Havens, R. A. (2005) The wisdom of Milton H. Erickson, CARMARTHAN: Crown House Publishing.

Kroger, W. S. and Fezler, W. D. (1976) Hypnosis and behaviour modification, MICHIGAN:J. B. Lippincott.

Moll, A. (2004) Hypnotism, MONTANA: Kessinger Publishing Co.

Marshall, P. (2012) Introduction to psychology, MANCHESTER: Oakley Books.

Marshall, P. (2012)b Understanding human memory, MANCHESTER: Oakley Books.

Marshall, P. (2012)c Unlocking your potential, MANCHESTER: Oakley Books.

Marshall, P. (2012)e How to study and learn, MANCHESTER: Oakley Books.

Marshall, P. (2012)f Improving your memory, MANCHESTER: Oakley Books.

Marshall, P. (2012)g Maximising your memory, MANCHESTER: Oakley Books.

Block, G. J. (1981), ed. Mesmerism: A translation of the original medical and scientific writings of F.A. Mesmer, CA: Kaufmann .

Robertson, D. (2009) ed. The discovery of hypnosis: The complete writings of James Braid the father of hypnotherapy, YORK: National Council for Hypnotherapy.

Salter, A. (2001) Conditioned reflex therapy, WA: Wellness Institute.

Selye, H. (1955) "Stress and disease". Science, Oct. 7, 1955; 122: 625-631.

Stanton, W. J. (1981) Fundamentals of marketing,, 6th. Edition, NY: McGraw-Hill.

Warwick, L, ed. (2012) Willings Press Guide), LONDON: Cision.

Wolinsky, S. (2007) Trances people live, NJ: Bramble Books.

Index

151

HOW TO STUDY AND LEARN
Your practical guide to effective study skills
Dr Peter Marshall

Are you thinking of studying or training for an important qualification? Do you know the best techniques for studying and learning to ensure you achieve the best results as quickly as possible? Whether you are at college or university, doing projects or assignments, writing essays, receiving continuous assessment or preparing for exams this is the book for you. Now in its third edition, this practical book covers getting your thinking right, organising yourself properly, finding and processing the information you need, reading effectively, developing good writing skills, thinking creatively, motivating yourself, and more. Whatever your subject, age or background, start now and turn yourself into a winning candidate.

UNLOCKING YOUR POTENTIAL
How to master your mind, life and destiny
Dr Peter Marshall

If you really want to unlock your potential and become master of your own life, you will need to remove the barriers to success, including your own narrow expectations and those imposed by others. This book will introduce you to techniques for overcoming the limiting effects of past conditioning, misguided or obsolete teachings and repressed conflicts. You will learn how to develop your creativity, improve your ability to solve problems and manage your social contacts to facilitate success.

MAXIMISING YOUR MEMORY
How to train yourself to remember more
Dr Peter Marshall

A powerful memory brings obvious advantages in educational, career and social terms. At school and college those certificates that provide a passport to a career depend heavily on what you can remember in the exam room. In the world of work, being able to recall details which slip the minds of colleagues will give you a competitive edge. In addition, one of the secrets of being popular with customers and friends is to remember their names and the little things that make them feel they matter to you. This popular book, now in its second edition, explains clearly how you can maximise your memory in order to achieve your academic, professional and personal goals.

UNDERSTANDING HUMAN MEMORY
What it is and how it Works
Dr Peter Marshall

This book explores the subject of human memory in all its dimensions – how it works physiologically and chemically, how it develops by conditioning and training, how it sometimes plays tricks on us to protect us, how it can fail through physiological damage and what we can do if it does. Now in its second edition, it will be essential reading for students of psychology, nursing, medicine and other disciplines concerned with understanding and management of human behaviour.

RESEARCH METHODS
How to choose and use the right methods
Dr Peter Marshall

All social science courses offered at universities or colleges include a research methods module, for which students are expected to purchase a research methods book. These are invariably weighty and expensive at a time when student funds are stretched. Dr Marshall has produced a reader-friendly, plain English and value-for-money solution. In this second edition, he explains the various methods available to social researchers and the basic principles, strengths and weakness involved in the use of both quantitative and qualitative methods. Whether you are new to the subject or an established practitioner this book should prove valuable. Dr Marshall has had many years experience in research and teaching in universities and colleges

IMPROVING YOUR MEMORY
The unique 5 x 5 system
Dr Peter Marshall

In the 21st century people live on their wits. What determines how successful they are in whatever they do is their mental ability and, to a large extent, that depends on their memory quality. The author and colleagues of London University discovered that memory quality has even replaced IQ as the dominant predictor of school outcomes. Deriving from such research, this book, now in its third edition, contains a powerful system for enhancing memory quality. Written in plain, concise language, it is simple, effective and comprehensive in its application. It has been tested over and over again on the young, the old, the bright and the not so bright and it can be mastered in just 7 – 10 hours.

EDUCATING A GIFTED CHILD
A guide for parents and teachers
Dr Peter Marshall

It is generally accepted today, and also UK government policy, that educational authorities must make provision for meeting the needs of gifted children. But how should they go about it? There is so much lack of agreement about what is the best strategy, about how to identify the gifted youngsters and even about what the concept of giftedness means. The author is a leading expert, who holds a doctorate from Manchester University in this subject. In plain English, in a balanced way and in a logical order, he covers everything a teacher, or a parent needs to know to meet the challenge of educating a gifted child.

INTRODUCTION TO PSYCHOLOGY
An introduction to exploring and understanding human behaviour
Dr Peter Marshall

Psychology can be a bewildering subject of study – so many theories, so much factual knowledge to acquire. This book makes a really great starting point for newcomers to the subject. Rather than just presenting lumps of psychological knowledge, it will teach you the skill of thinking like a psychologist. Never again will you be stuck for something worthwhile to say in a tutorial or to add value to an essay. Whether you are an undergraduate, A-level student or open access student, this student-friendly companion, now in its second edition, will set you on the right path.

For more information about this author go to:
https://www.amazon.com/author/drpetermarshall